To Chris and Lynn,

10/11/11.

KT-145-694

Finding
Harmony

With Best Wishes

Sally Wheeler

SALLY HYDER

Finding Harmony

The remarkable dog that helped
a family through the darkest of times

HARPER

HARPER

An Imprint of HarperCollins*Publishers*
77–85 Fulham Palace Road
Hammersmith, London W6 8JB

www.harpercollins.co.uk

First published in Great Britain by HarperCollins*Publishers* 2011

1 3 5 7 9 10 8 6 4 2

A catalogue record for this book is
available from the British Library

ISBN 978-0-00-739358-9

Printed and bound in Great Britain by
Clays Ltd, St Ives plc

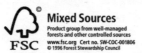

Mixed Sources
Product group from well-managed
forests and other controlled sources
www.fsc.org   Cert no. SW-COC-001806
© 1996 Forest Stewardship Council

FSC is a non-profit international organisation established to promote the
responsible management of the world's forests. Products carrying the FSC
label are independently certified to assure consumers that they come
from forests that are managed to meet the social, economic and
ecological needs of present and future generations.

Find out more about HarperCollins and the environment at
www.harpercollins.co.uk/green

To Andrew, without whom no mountains
would have been climbed and to Peter, Clara
and Melissa who have had their own mountains
to climb. And of course to Harmony, who has
opened doors to independence.
I love you.
Thank you.

Prologue

I've fallen in love with Elmo – at least I think I have. I've come to meet the new batch of dogs; they're only 12 months old. It's one of those bright January days and the barn is flush with sunlight. Here come Caesar and Elmo, old hands looking for new partners, and Headley, a choco-late Labrador who likes to watch me very carefully with his enormous brown eyes. I'm humbled by his trust. Then there are the blondes: Foster, who doesn't like 'boarding school' (as I have dubbed the advance training), still goes home to a foster family at night. Harry and Henry who I can't tell apart (Harry, I think, has the edge) are full of beans while Harmony is smaller and paler than the rest, with schoolgirl freckles on her face.

Having worked on the simplest tasks such as retriev-ing dropped items or just walking around without knocking into each other, we're now practising the super-market checkout sequence. The idea is for your dog to retrieve cans and boxes from the shelves, put them in your basket and then pass your purse to the checkout person. It's complicated: already I've run over a couple of paws with my wheelchair. There was an outburst of yelps.

'Sorry!' I exclaimed, mortified.

'Don't worry,' said the dog trainers, who have the patience of saints.

They check the dogs' paws, reassuring me. We reach the checkout counter in the corner of the barn – it looks exactly like the real thing.

'Go through,' I say, rehearsing the commands. 'Back, back, *back*!'

After releasing another foot of lead, I wait for Elmo to go backwards, facing me, past the counter. Hand high, I instruct him to take my purse and he grips it between his teeth.

'Up table, give it to the lady!' I tell him.

He puts his front paws on the table and hands it over to Claire, who is playing the checkout girl.

'Off!' I say, then again, 'Up table, get the purse. Bring it here!'

Elmo follows the commands with immense patience but I feel frazzled. This is so complicated: will I ever get it right? Will the trainers think I'm useless and unable to manage a dog?

'Good dog,' I tell him. I reach into the treat bag and find a bit of sausage. Elmo gently takes it from me, wagging his tail. In fact, the dogs wag their tails the whole time as if they're happy to be working. I pat his coat and I'm reminded not to stroke the top of his head. (How would you like it if a stranger patted the top of *your* head?)

Prologue

It doesn't take a rocket scientist to discover how to get a dog to work for you – rewards. As Canine Partners (a disability charity now in its twentieth year that uses specially trained dogs to assist people in their everyday lives) will tell you, there are lots of reasons why dogs won't work for you: too tired, hungry, hot, bored ... But there are two reasons why they want to do so: rewards and fun. My reward bag is full of chopped cheese, sausage, broccoli and carrot (yes, dogs eat vegetables too!). Every time I stick my hand in, I think, *yuck! Do I really have to live with a bag of mushy treats attached to me forever?*

'Keep rewarding,' says Claire, the trainer. 'Turn off your chair whenever you're stationary.'

So many things to remember: the last time I was here, I worked with Claire's dog, Doyle. Doyle is a Standard Poodle Retriever Cross (or 'Goldiepoo', as they are sometimes called). He works as a demo dog all the time. *Here we go again*, I could see him thinking as I dropped my purse on the floor. *Yeah, yeah, I know I have to pick it up!* He looked at me, big sigh, and then picked it up. I worked with Doyle after teaming up with Guy, a high-spirited Flat Coat. After trying to manage Guy, I felt exhausted – Doyle was a dream in comparison.

At lunch, Claire asks: 'Do you have a preference?'

'Elmo and Headley,' I reply, without hesitation.

'What about Harmony?'

'She's too quiet,' I insist. 'Too docile – boring, even: I want a dog with real character.'

In the afternoon we're sent out to exercise the dogs, one at a time, in a field at the back. They tear across the frozen ground. I wrap my scarf around my neck and throw the ball (supplied by a local tennis club) for Foster. He brings it back and drops it in my lap. Ears cocked, he stares at me. *Come on lady, what are you waiting for?* I throw the ball again and again and again. All of a sudden, I realise it's going to be fun as well as useful, having one of these dogs.

'Do you recognise who this is?'

It's Becca, the head trainer. She walks towards me with a dog: Harmony. I smile. She takes Foster indoors. Harmony races over, making a sound I later learn to associate with happiness, a mix of a purr and a growl. She places her paws on my lap. Can she really be that pleased to see me? I'm flattered. Vicky, another trainer, lets me get on with it but I feel reassured by the knowledge that she's still there and ready to step in, if I need her.

I know what I'm expected to do … I throw the ball.

Harmony brings it back.

Then she runs off without the ball and I watch her sniffing the hedgerows and chasing her shadow. I love her curiosity. As I observe her, unnoticed, I feel strangely peaceful. Something in me clicks: *I might have been wrong about Harmony*. Then she sneezes. Startled by the sound of her own sneeze, she bolts across the field. Her excitement is infectious; I start laughing and can't stop. I drive the disability scooter as fast as I can all over the field. It goes much faster than the one at home and Harmony tears after me; we weave in and out of each other. I feel the wind on my face and in my hair; I've smiled so much my teeth have gone dry.

Prologue

I've remembered what it was to *want* to be outdoors in the fresh air, trudging through muddy fields, hill walking, climbing mountains and reaching North Everest Base Camp.

Oh, do we have to stop?

Then Harmony decides to let me know she's there and comes bounding over. I lift her face to reach mine. She nuzzles into my neck and I see the brown streaks behind her ears: it's as if she's tried to apply self-tanning lotion and made a mess of it. She's tried to smooth it on but it's trickled down her body and legs, and then dried. On her forehead she has a 'fingerprint' – a spot just perfect for kissing. Her tail curves backwards and wags furiously; I feel my heart reach out to her. *She's slow to respond to commands, she's going to need lots of encouragement but there's something special in there*, I think to myself.

I've taken to this little soul.

1

In the Beginning

As you approach it, Everest gets bigger: you don't appreciate the scale of it until you leave the last of the Tibetan villages clinging to the mountainside, the prayer flags fluttering in the breeze. Gleaming white against a big blue sky she is majestic – no wonder the Tibetans call her *Qomolungma* (Goddess Mother of the World).

Our journey to Everest began before we reached Tibet: it started when Andrew, my then boyfriend of six years, decided he wanted to celebrate passing his BSc in Estate Management at Reading University by going on a big trip.

'Let's take three months off before I start work,' he suggested, one night after supper. 'Let's do a proper trip. Wouldn't you love to see China? How about Tibet?'

Andrew and I have been together since he was 18 and I was 20. None of this would have happened without him. He's a very private person, but it would be unfair to go on without acknowledging this is our story: we've always been a team.

We met in Edinburgh in 1979, when I was 17 while I was studying drama. One bleak Sunday morning in

Finding Harmony

January, a year into my course, I heard singing coming from a local neighbourhood church and went in. Raised by, then, agnostic parents, I had no experience of going to church other than attending the local youth club, which was run by the Baptist church in the village in Fife where I grew up. There, the emphasis was on fun, not God. But I'm a very emotional person with a love of choral music: I went in, sat down and by the end of the service, I was elated.

Through the church I met a wonderful group of people who welcomed me into their congregation. The first person I met was Reg, an elderly man who took the time to make sure that I was sitting with people of my own age. Also, there were families who would invite me to join them for Sunday lunch and gave me lifts to and from church.

A few months later, I met Andrew. He was taking part in a playlet: a dialogue between God (a girl in the pulpit) and Man (Andrew at the prayer lectern). My first thought was, *I haven't seen you before*. This was quickly followed by: *I want to get to know you*. When we finally spoke, he came across as a real gentleman. He has a lovely smile and the biggest brown eyes you've ever seen; he also has incredibly long eyelashes. Women die for them! He's dark and handsome with, I found out much later, an Indian great-grandfather. Andrew was mature for his age with an articulacy that meant he could express things in a word, usually *yes*, whereas I'd use about twenty. I felt able to express myself freely and be understood. It was something I'd been searching for, I realised. He was non-judgemental and a great listener.

In the Beginning

We soon discovered a shared belief in working hard, enjoying life and giving back to society by looking after folk less fortunate than ourselves. After three years at drama school, studying works such as George Bernard Shaw's *Arms and the Man* and Shakespeare's *Macbeth*; also putting on productions of J. M. Synge's *The Playboy of the Western World* and Federico Garcia Lorca's *Blood Wedding,* I decided acting wasn't for me. I wasn't enough of a performer to pursue it as a profession and so toyed with the idea of studying drama therapy but needed a psychiatric nurse qualification first. So my thoughts turned to nursing. At drama school I'd learned the art of public speaking and appearing self-confident. So, in November 1983 I joined the RMN course at the Royal Infirmary of Edinburgh which, at the time was based in a collection of old buildings with turrets and spiral stair-cases in the heart of the city. I did a placement on a medi-cal ward (oncology) and I loved it. Once there, I made great friends and immediately knew it was for me although I had to work hard to convince the tutors this was a genuine decision, that I really wanted to care for cancer sufferers. I qualified as a general nurse in February 1987.

For Andrew and myself commitment and loyalty to each other and the things we did, our jobs and now of course our family feature high on our list of priorities. We are also very different: to this day, for example, I still don't know which party Andrew votes for – a long time ago we agreed not to discuss politics. Some things remain a mystery: how can anyone take or leave chocolate, for example? I once found an eight-year-old Mars Bar in his rucksack that had formed part of his emergency rations. Personally, I can't be within a 100-yard radius of chocolate without having to eat it all. I am impulsive whereas Andrew thinks things through very carefully; I'm noisy and a chatterbox while he is quiet and deep yet we both love books, good food and climbing mountains.

Now, by climbing I'm not talking about ropes and crampons (attachments to outdoor footwear). I briefly joined the Edinburgh University mountaineering club only to discover that I loved abseiling down, but hated going up! No, I'm talking about hill walking. My childhood in Fife instilled a passion for walking. 'Munro-bagging', they call it in Scotland: a term used to describe going up the 283 Munro Mountains (Ben Nevis being the most famous) that Mr Munro mapped in the nineteenth century.

As a child of the Sixties, Munro-bagging was a regular weekend pursuit. I rarely watched TV although I'll never forget being woken up to witness Neil Armstrong take one giant leap for mankind.

'This is important and you need to remember it,' insisted Dad, bundling me downstairs.

On Saturdays, my father worked an extra job selling carpets and would come home with sweets, stories of difficult customers and newly hatched sales pitches. Meanwhile, I spent many a happy afternoon in the local farmers' fields 'tatty scouring'. All the kids did it: clearing the fields after the tractor had pulled up the potatoes, proudly bringing home bags of spuds for our mums.

Sundays, however, were reserved for walking. After breakfast, Mum, Dad and I would set off, with Dad in socks and boots, whatever the weather. 'No good comes of baring your feet,' he used to say, me in my Dunlop Green Flash. I have photos of us in hand-crocheted multi-coloured waistcoats and memories of trudging up hills in orange bell-bottoms, with embroidered flowers swinging round my ankles. Real seventies' flair! Days were filled with the sound of our breath, the crunch of footsteps, rucksacks loaded with Marmite and cottage cheese sand-wiches plus flasks of sweet tea. Although I didn't think about it at the time (I wished then that I had parents who didn't march up and down hills), it was there that I discovered my love of silence and being alone with your thoughts – it's all part of the joy and discipline of climbing.

We walked up to the Old Man of Storr on the Isle of Skye and ate our lunch watching the clouds come in. It was snowing on the way down. When I was 16, we walked the Cuillin ridge from Sligachan, up and over to Loch Coruisk. Increasingly reluctantly, I followed Dad to the top. I stopped early, but he came back for me.

'Come on, Sally. It's not far to the top. Believe me, it's worth it!' he insisted.

As we reached the lip and looked out, it was then that I understood how you *earn* a view. The challenge of the climb is rewarded by the achievement of reaching the summit, then seeing the landscape open out before you.

Just before Christmas 1986, Andrew surprised me with the news that we were going hiking, abroad.

'Morocco,' he announced, after perusing the travel section of the local bookstore over the course of a few weeks. 'Walking in the Anti Atlas Mountains. What do you think?'

I couldn't wait.

Feeling that it would be safer to travel to North Africa in a group rather than doing it alone, we booked our trip through an organised group called Explore Worldwide. The next gruelling six months saw me sitting my Final nursing exams and working in the oncology unit again. That December we flew into Marrakech with a bunch of 10 Brits. My first taste of the exotic, it was love at first sight. Entranced, Andrew and I wandered through the *souks*, a maze of alleyways where you could buy red clay for staining lips, henna and believe it or not, second-hand false teeth! We bartered for a sheepskin and watched pet monkeys swing from men's shoulders. At night the main square came alive with fire-eaters and snake charmers, tarot-readers and storytellers. We ate spicy butterbean stew from wooden bowls and absorbed the Arabic voices and foreign smells. I made a point of looking at the women (whose faces were hidden in burkas) in the eye. If I smiled and nodded, so did they. Otherwise they formed a silent counterpart to their men.

On Christmas Eve we took the bus through the Tiz 'n' Test Pass, leaving the mountains behind in a cloud of orange dust. Christmas was spent in the blistering-hot desert town of Taroudant. The hotel's palm tree had cotton wool stuck to its leaves and we drank beer from bottles decorated with pictures of Father Christmas. Our seven-course lunch on the day itself consisted of spam fritters, potatoes, salad, soup, burnt chicken, processed peas and cake, served separately and in that order, much to our amusement. The next day was spent walking in the mountains. Escape from the heat (we were on the border of the Sahara) into the cool mountain air was a welcome relief. In the distance we could make out an oasis of palms and orange groves; beyond was desert, stretching as far as the eye could see.

For a week, we roamed the mountains and all sorts of crazy adventures befell us. We stayed in lots of different villages, once in an old derelict house with no running water or electricity. We ate by candlelight and I was given a *djellaba* (a long, loose-fitting robe) that I wore as we listened to the splash of rain by an open fire while the men played homemade musical instruments, mostly drums but some whistle- and flute-like ones too. Of course no other women were present, but I loved sitting and communicating with the villagers, exchanging ideas about children and marriage through signs and gestures (no one spoke English). In the fishing village of Essaouira, Cat Stevens (remember him?) gave the Call to Prayer at 6.30am and we discovered the joy of eating barbecued sweetcorn and fresh sardines. When it was eventually time to go home, Andrew and I were both thinking the same thing: *There is so much out there.*

A door had opened and we could see what lay ahead: the big wide world.

* * *

Finding Harmony

The only problem with Scotland in 1987 was unemployment. Although I'd qualified there as a nurse, in the end I had to move down to London to find a job. It wasn't too much of a sacrifice, though, as Andrew was by then studying Estate Management in Reading. On 14 February, I reported for duty on the general medical ward at Guy's, a big teaching hospital not far from London Bridge. I moved into a single room on site. It was a hovel – hot and noisy, with the sounds of trains and the pub and all the other resident nurses in their rooms. The kitchen was disgusting, but Andrew bought me a slow cooker, perfect for stews and soups. It's still in use today.

I hated the smell of London in the summer: the metallic tang on your tongue, dog poo on the pavements and vegetables rotting in the sun, the sludge of the Thames. Luckily, I didn't have to wait long before I was moved to a shared flat, newly built and also on site. At my request I was transferred to the oncology unit, where I was responsible for caring for hundreds of patients in an L-shaped ward; men down one side and women down the other, bone-marrow transplants in the side rooms, chemotherapy everywhere. At weekends, Andrew would come up and we spent happy days together (when I was lucky enough to be off-duty) walking through the city, queuing for stand-by tickets at the Globe and going to West End musicals. We loved the musicals: our favourites then were *Starlight Express* and *Les Misérables* but we also enjoyed *Cats* and later on, *The Phantom of the Opera* (you might say we were suckers for anything Andrew Lloyd Webber cared to throw our way!).

In the Beginning

Memories of those productions have stayed with us. Andrew and Clara have also done the West End shows and being musical, sing the songs at the tops of their voices. It's lovely to think we've managed to pass on our appreciation to the next generation.

For those brief, fun-packed months, London felt like our city.

Then I began to feel unwell.

The first acute symptom was a pain in my side. This was in the March, just after I'd arrived in the City and started work at Guy's. At first, I'd felt lonely but now I also felt scared. The symptoms worsened: I needed pethidine to control the pain, breathing was difficult, my chest and abdomen began to ache and I was running a fever. Concerned, the doctors eventually diagnosed Bornholm Disease (named after the islands of Bornholm in Denmark) and caused by a coxsackie – group B common virus – that inflames the intercostal muscles. I was admitted to the hospital I worked in, a very strange experience indeed. Being new in town I knew hardly anyone but the staff that I worked with came to visit me and my new flatmates moved my stuff to the flat.

After a week I was discharged and went to recuperate at Uncle Andrew (my mother's brother) and Aunty Pat's home in St Neots, Cambridgeshire. They were extremely kind and pulled me through. I remember watching the Zeebrugge disaster on the television: a car ferry capsized just outside the Belgian port killing hundreds, which added to my sense of mortality. I focused on getting back to work and making a full recovery.

Finding Harmony

Eventually, I arrived back in time for a hot London summer and the slog of working on the wards but I never seemed to improve, not properly: I felt dizzy and exhausted all the time. In the end, Andrew and I decided that I needed a proper break and so I took unpaid leave. That August, we flew to Vancouver for our next foreign adventure.

Aunty Margaret and Uncle Gary (family on my father's side) had a beef ranch in Mayerthorpe, Alberta. They lived there with their three daughters (Helen, Jennifer and Sandra) and one son (Richard); one of my cousins and her husband has since taken over the farm. In 1966, Margaret went out to Canada on a government-sponsored scheme designed to attract more radiographers to the country. There, she met my Uncle Gary, whose pioneering family had created a farm out of the wilderness. On finding they were short of labour, we spent two very happy weeks working on the farm: Andrew drove the tractor and grew a beard while I helped to pickle dill from the garden, picked fruit and vegetables and took lunch to the men working in the fields in a pail. I was Laura Ingalls Wilder in *Little House on the Prairie*! Tanned and restored by our outdoor life and with the chirping of crickets and fields of wheat blowing in the wind, we said our goodbyes and hitched our way across the Rockies to Montreal.

We took in the Niagara Falls, ate stacks of diner pancakes dripping with maple syrup (the coffee was undrinkable) and soaked up the sense of space offered by those monumental Canadian landscapes. At this point, we also learned the rules of hitch hiking.

In the Beginning

'Never throw your bags in the boot,' warned the driver of a truck complete with double bed and fridge who took pity on us and feared for our safety after I climbed into the front seat, leaving Andrew to do the bags. 'I could have driven off with the bags and left you behind!'

Lesson learned.

Six weeks later, back in London we realised that we had caught the travelling bug. Now the city seemed more claustrophobic than ever but no sooner had we returned to our working and student lives than Andrew was revisiting the travel sections of local bookstores and eagerly planning our next trip.

2

Surprise on Everest

In the summer of 1988 Andrew passed his exams, New Order's 'Blue Monday' was back in the charts and Melanie Griffith, the ultimate eighties' poster-girl, was out-manoeuvring male colleagues in *Working Girl*. We were off again. On a hot Saturday afternoon in June we caught the Tube to Trailfinders, the Holy Grail for travellers on London's Kensington High Street, where we purchased air tickets into Hong Kong and out of Delhi. It was the journey we had been building up to: first Canada and Morocco, now Asia.

'It's my responsibility to show you this,' said the travel agent, passing us a copy of a warning issued by the Foreign Office:

Customers have been advised of a volatile situation between arrival and departure points.

'So, travelling between China and India isn't officially recommended?' asked Andrew.

'Not *officially*,' said the travel agent.

'Oh well,' I smiled.

Tickets in hand, we walked over to Holland Park for a celebration picnic, at which point Andrew turned into a magician. Instead of pulling rabbits out of a top hat, he produced from his rucksack a tablecloth, glasses, champagne and smoked salmon. It was the most ridiculously romantic gesture I'd ever seen and perfectly suited to the white-walled gardens, the sunshine and our elated mood.

Later that week Andrew came home with a shiny copy of *The Lonely Planet Guide to China* and we spent hours poring over photographs of the Great Wall of China and figuring out our route. First, though, we had to earn the fare. Earlier that year I had decided that I wanted to care for the terminally ill and had been offered a place at St Christopher's Hospice in Sydenham, Kent. I'd realised that the part of the oncology job that I found most rewarding was when the battle and stress of chemotherapy and radiotherapy were over and palliative care was the way forward; it was a more positive and holistic way to be with the patients, I wanted to get to know them, to treat them as individuals and I was keen to learn how to do this type of specialist nursing in what was then the best place in the UK for palliative medicine.

I'd decided to defer my new challenge until Andrew had finished his BSc, so I went back to Guy's. That spring was spent working as a nurse from 7.30 until 3pm before rushing across London to a smoky wine-bar near Price Waterhouse in the Embankment. There, I changed into a black dress and white apron, then popped champagne corks for pink-faced city boys, who gave me 10 per cent of their tabs – the tips were insane. I was there until 8pm every night. Otherwise days and nights off were spent working as an agency nurse in private hospitals all over London. Officially this was 'moonlighting' but there was such a shortage of nurses then that it was easy to get extra work and everyone did it. I worked hard that spring, but it was worth it.

Eventually, it was time to go. Sometimes when I look back on our trip through China, I wonder, how did we know which trains to catch? No one spoke English. We went prepared: we had the usual jabs – cholera, typhoid and Hepatitis B – and bought bags of malaria tablets. Also, we took our own chopsticks (a precaution because of the risk of Hepatitis B) and had rabies vaccines, which can buy you a bit of time if you're bitten by a dog. In Tibet, if you fail as a monk then you come back as a dog, which accounts for the packs of wild dogs in the temples (nothing to do with the food left lying around, of course). Although we didn't voice our hopes for fear of disappointment, secretly both of us harboured the same dream of seeing the Potala Palace in Lhasa, the former home of the Dalai Lama.

We woke up on the descent into Hong Kong after a night flight. The plane flew so close to the skyscrapers that you could see what people were eating for breakfast! Its wheels hit the ground, it braked before tipping into the sea, the doors opened and we were met by a wall of heat.

What a shock.

We found a room in Kowloon on the mainland. A fairly grotty place. We were kept up by the all-night chatter, doors slamming and general commotion. The next morning I woke up with 25 tick bites. Things improved when we found the Youth Hostel on top of the hill on Hong Kong Island. Its whitewashed buildings were a refuge from the hustle and bustle of downtown Hong Kong and there was a strong sea breeze.

We spent our first days wandering through the streets and stalls, marvelling at the strangeness of it all, in particular the food. I am fairly sure we accidentally ended up eating animal intestines but somehow survived. After securing our Chinese visas, we caught the overnight ferry to China's mainland: to Guangzhou, as the City of Canton was then known. Everywhere we went the Chinese were fascinated by my blonde hair, which caused quite a sensation. Women would approach with out-stretched arms to touch it and I'd usually oblige. Our rucksacks were also an innovation: they beat straw ropes, which was what the Chinese used to carry everything.

Certain things we figured out pretty quickly. When you arrive in a new place, buy a ticket out immediately (demand is high). We always went hard sleeper, too. Each carriage had 20 rows of three-tiered bunks – the secret was to go for middle and bottom. If you got the top bunk, you were squashed against the ceiling where tiny fans whirred day and night. On our first journey, I opened the window to let air in and a Chinese man shut it. I opened it again. Wrong! This was a steam train and the smoke and soot blew straight in our eyes; it was even worse going through a tunnel. Those 33-hour journeys were long, with people spitting and vendors offering fried food through open windows at the stations.

But there was plenty to marvel at: light flooded the valleys and the endless green paddy fields. In fact, there was a strange tranquillity in the knowledge that you couldn't go anywhere but just had to sit there with all those people and the train jolting beneath you and take it all in. It's amazing how the mind can release its normal grip on time when you allow it to do so.

Suddenly a group of Chinese women appeared and motioned for me to accompany them. I got up and followed them down the train, where I found Laura, an English girl, in floods of tears. She was going to Shanghai for her medical elective. Overwhelmed by the foreignness and loneliness of it all, as well as her predicament, she couldn't stop weeping. Alarmed, her fellow passengers had gone in search of other foreigners known to be travelling on the train. Laura cheered up when she saw me and shared her fears. How lucky I was, I realised, to have Andrew. I sat comparing travel notes with Laura until we parted at Shanghai, by which stage she was once again looking forward to her adventure.

From Shanghai our journey took us up the Yangtze River in a decrepit old passenger boat. It was filthy, with squatting toilets and inedible food (if you were lucky enough to find any) and was as hot as a furnace. We'd booked second-class tickets and found ourselves stuffed into an airless, crowded dormitory but then we met a couple of English tourists who had cleverly booked a first-class cabin with curtains and a breeze. Instantly, we became best friends and took refuge in their cabin, playing cards and chatting.

We disembarked at Nanjing and then went on to Xian to see the newly discovered Terracotta Army. Standing in a vast cavern, looking at those mythical soldiers was a surprisingly moving experience.

It was becoming increasingly apparent that the authorities didn't like independent travellers. We had to keep avoiding the CITS (Chinese International Travel Service), who were keen to bus everyone to the foreigners' hotels, where they could keep tabs on us all. Instead we stayed at a student hostel in Beijing University, where everyone wanted to talk to us. *Big things are going to happen*, we were told. We had no idea what the students meant but the following year, 1989, came the Tiananmen Square massacre. You could see the curiosity and interest in the young people's faces as they asked questions about the other side of the globe, places they could only dream of. We felt like early travellers coming back with reports of life in faraway countries: we were the lucky ones.

From Beijing we travelled out to the Ming Tombs and the Great Wall of China. Within moments of walking, we found ourselves alone, gazing out at mountains that seemed to be forever rolling on; the scale was incredible. The Great Wall snakes into the distance and I can well believe that it can be seen from space.

And all the time we dreamed of Tibet.

But we weren't the only ones. The closer we got to the border, the more Westerners we met, all intent on making the same journey. 'Have you noticed beer is cheaper than bottled water?' was a common greeting. There was a sense of camaraderie among the Europeans which meant we operated as one: we were tourists from the same place – the West. We arrived in Xinning and then went onto Golmud, the end of the railway line, which resembled a film-set of dusty nothingness. It was an eerie place. Behind us the sun disappeared in clouds of dust and I fell horribly ill after eating a yak burger. Lying in the hotel bed, thinking I was about to die, I became obsessed with a need for apple juice.

'I want apple juice!' I moaned.

When Andrew appeared through the door, hours later, with a tin can of fizzy apple juice, I thought I was hallucinating. Gulping it down thirstily, I felt instantly better.

By the time we arrived in Golmud we were among a group of 10 Westerners from Canada, USA, Switzerland and the UK – a big bunch of backpackers. We were herded into a hotel by the notorious CITS, who told us we would have to pay £200 each for a three-day trip into Tibet – 'guided', of course. As we wanted to travel through Tibet and on into Nepal this represented a bit of an issue, never mind the cost. After discovering one of our group spoke Tibetan, we could scarcely believe our luck. Now we could improvise: we could smuggle ourselves over the border, which was exactly what we did.

Serendipity has a funny way of taking over in situations like this. You just need to know roughly where to look and be prepared to pay for it. Before long, we had found a local bus driver who was driving the scheduled bus long distance into Tibet. We were smuggled out of the hotel in the middle of night when it was pitch-black. At the Chinese checkpoint where we left Golmud, the driver turned off the bus lights.

No one spoke English.

It was real cloak-and-dagger stuff: we were disguised in cowboy hats and cloaks provided by the Tibetans. The biggest problem was my blonde hair, which I had to stuff inside my hat. When the bus stopped we were herded out to walk around potholes too deep for it to be driven across, some stretching 20 feet long. We were conscious of passengers being beaten by Chinese soldiers but no one asked why.

Then we passed into Lhasa.

'Not in China now, no passports,' the hostel keeper informed us.

Grinning from ear to ear, we dumped our bags on the floor. We'd made it, though we weren't entirely sure how it had happened.

The next morning – a crystal-clear day – we woke up in Lhasa and gazed up at the Palace, which sits on a ridge and was framed by the mountain range with slopes of snow and rock. It was as if we'd stepped back in time. We got dressed, had some tea and went for a walk. In silence, we gazed up at the *stupas* containing the bodies of all the Dalai Llamas.

'Psssst!'

We turned to find a young monk behind a pillar.

'You speak English?' he asked (it was illegal for Tibetans to learn English).

'Yes.'

He showed us a book.

'AD,' he said. 'What does this mean?'

'Anno Domini, the year of our Lord. Have you heard of Christ?'

His face lit up: 'Ah, the Pope!'

Although we always hoped to get to Tibet, the prospect of climbing the Everest Foothills had been a distant reality. It only began to sink in as we packed our rucksacks with supplies for the trip. I've got a photo of Andrew sitting on the bed in the guesthouse studying the guidebook. Beside him on a wooden table is a pile of cans and packets, the tallest stack being noodles. (In the high altitude, the water wouldn't boil and we had to eat them still crunchy.) Next to the noodles are cans of spam, lychees, peas, a jar of redcurrant jam, powdered baby milk that we drank with melted chocolate squares on top (delicious!), *sampa* (barley rolled in yak milk to make little balls of dough like a solid porridge) and loo rolls. We had to buy it all from the Friendship Store (a store only foreigners can use) as nothing was available locally. It meant playing along with the Chinese, using their currency rather than the local Tibetan Riminbi and pretending we were just tourists there for the day.

It's amazing to think this is what got us up 5,208 metres, along with Andrew's quiet insistence.

'Come on, Sally. Just a little bit further!'

After a few days in Lhasa, during which time the big Nepal earthquake had injured more than 16,000 people

– and we ourselves felt the tremors – we caught the local bus to Gyantse. When the driver tried to overtake a lorry on a hairpin bend, I found myself sitting above the rear wheel as it spun over emptiness. I let out a loud scream.

'Try not to let your imagination run away with you,' advised Andrew, the voice of calm.

The driver accelerated hard enough to send the truck hurtling forward, away from the precipice and on into Gyantse. From there, we hitched a ride west to Tingri, lying flat in the open back of a lorry like fugitives. It was exciting, even though the journey seemed to take forever. Every so often the driver would stop, enjoy a few more bottles of beer and gamble with the householders who had provided the refreshment. Arriving with blackened faces from the exhaust, safe but sore, we felt like real adventurers now.

'Come on, Sally. Just a bit further!'

The aim was to get to Rombuk monastery. At 5,000 metres above sea level, it's the highest monastery in the world. By now we were a group of seven. Together, we hired a couple of yaks and a guide and stayed in yak-skin tents, which have a hole in the top to allow smoke from the yak-dung fires to escape. We drank yak tea (or 'yuck tea', as it came to be known). Made from tea, salt and yak butter, unless drunk very quickly it congeals on your tongue. The climb was slow and hard work; we all suffered forms of mild altitude sickness but one of our group actually had to go back as he was clearly unwell and the only cure is to descend. At one stage we had to cross a roaring river via a crumbling stone bridge that I was convinced would collapse beneath our weight. Otherwise, there was just silence and fluttering prayer flags, the rumble of prayer wheels (wooden wheels reputed to accumulate wisdom and good karma as they spin) and the occasional flap of bird wings. It's a desert region: food is hard to come by and there is no green, just mile upon mile of rocks and Everest shrouded in mist in the distance, drawing us ever closer.

Arriving at Rombuk monastery is unexpected: after a two-day walk up the valley, you turn a corner and the ridge flattens out. There it is, clinging to the side of the Everest valley like a beleaguered fortress. The monastery is still inhabited by a community of monks and nuns whose lives are dedicated to God and survival. With their lined, weathered faces and faded tunics, they seem to belong there on the mountainside. We stayed in a platform hut built on dried mud, with Tibetan rugs and the best loo with a view I've ever encountered. From there, you could see Her Majesty. The monks also operate an efficient black market currency exchange and charged an extortionate amount for their eggs, which just goes to show everyone has to survive somehow.

As soon as we arrived at the monastery, I looked at Andrew and knew from his set jaw and gleaming eyes that he'd decided to go on. Now the plan was to get to North Everest Base Camp: just seven kilometres of rocky terrain with heavily loaded rucksacks away. After a fitful night's sleep on a hard floor and more green tea, we set out the next morning.

'Just a bit further, Sally.'

CLICK!

I took a photo to remember the spot, the exhaustion and the sheer elation of being on top of the world (well, almost!). Here's Andrew in his Harris sweater knitted by my dad (we had one each) and walking boots. He looks every bit the gentleman explorer – no different, in fact, to George Mallory and Andrew Irvine, the first British mountaineers to attempt to scale Everest in the 1920s from the Tibetan side. Mallory gave the infamous answer to the question, 'Why did you climb it?': 'Because it's there.'

Only Andrew's white-framed sunglasses (oh, so eighties!) give the decade away.

We reached the British Base Camp in the afternoon. This turned out to be a bunch of scruffy huts and more prayer flags, looking ragged; there was a cairn and tents and provisions. I had expected posh tents but they didn't look any different to the ones we saw when walking the Munros. Yet despite the low-key nature of the camp, our moment of arrival still stands out as the most exhilarating of my life: to be there on the flanks of Everest (and not on the Nepalese side on a guided tour) and all down to our own initiative and resources was a remarkable feeling.

Unloading our rucksacks, we tried to take it all in. We were so close to Everest that the view was obscured by whiteness; it was hard to connect where we were with the myths and expectations surrounding the world's highest mountain – she was every bit as powerful as the place she holds in our imagination. *No wonder men sacrifice their lives for her*, I thought, cupping a hand over my eyes to avoid the glare.

I sat down.

'No, come on,' said Andrew. 'I want to go a bit further!'

'Right now?'

'Yes.'

I stood up.

'OK, that's far enough,' he said, half an hour later. 'I want a photograph of us with Everest in the background. Can you take a photo?' He gave the camera to our new friend Peter, a Canadian mountaineer. 'Actually, take loads!'

Andrew had taken off his ski-jacket. His lips were chapped and his nose, like mine, was striped with sunblock. He came and joined me in front of the camera. Together, we blinked in the sun and I relaxed into the pose. Then all of a sudden, he dropped down on one knee.

'*Andrew?*'

I watched him rummage in the camera case hanging from his neck then I looked over his shoulder towards the craggy face of Everest and its snow-covered slopes.

He can't have planned this in London.

'Will you marry me?'

I burst out laughing. As he pushed a diamond and ruby ring over my finger, I started to weep with happiness.

I had waited so long to be asked and now when I least expected his proposal and it couldn't have been further from my mind, there it was. Insane. In the space of a few hours, all my dreams were coming true. My next thought was, *get the ring back in that box before you lose it!*

'Yes,' I replied. '*Yes!*'

That night we celebrated our engagement at Base Camp with the British expedition teams who had failed to scale the Northeast ridge as the bad weather had come in. The men were tired and gruff. It felt so exciting to be there, eavesdropping on their stories, that I didn't appreciate how disappointed they must have felt at not succeeding. One of their group was part of the mountain rescue team in Glencoe and another belonged to the Guinness family. With them were the Sherpas, quite extraordinary men who get themselves and everyone else up Everest, carrying loads, while more often than not inadequately equipped or reliant on the teams to equip them. For me, it was a glimpse into a world I would never see again.

Meanwhile, I twisted my engagement ring round and round my finger. During the trip, I'd lost so much weight that my fingers had shrunk and it didn't fit: the ruby glinted, blood red, in the firelight. We drank whisky and ate the Scottish food provided for us by the team: tinned mince and peas followed by Dundee cake. After months of rice, the food was too rich and we were all violently sick.

Once I'd recovered, I called Mum on the UK team's satellite phone (there were no mobile phones in those days).

'Andrew's asked me to marry him.'

'What is the terminal moraine like?' came the reply.

Mum's a geography teacher – well, she was then – and she's crazy about mountains. My laughter echoed around the world, distorted by the thousands of miles between Tibet and Scotland. We spoke to Dad then rang Andrew's parents. All were relieved to hear from us and also happy with our news. The evening was as unexpected as life itself. We listened to the mountaineers' stories and felt blissfully tired and full of whisky.

I have a photograph of Andrew on bended knee and me in sunglasses, my hair in a ponytail, looking like the happiest couple on earth.

Next morning, the rest of the tourist group left Base Camp to begin their descent but we stayed put. The British expedition team lent us a tent. We wanted to celebrate our engagement and they, perhaps to alleviate their gloom, were happy to have us there. They were all a bit depressed: the anti-climax of failing to reach the summit after years of preparation and expectation must have been hard to bear. When it was time to leave, we thumbed a ride with the team to the main road. The truck driver was a maniac and the Sherpas jumped out of the back of the truck. I remember thinking, if they've jumped out we're entitled to be scared but there was no way we could escape.

We had planned to continue through to Nepal but the road was blocked due to the earthquake and so we ended up with a two-day drive, again hitched. Back in Lhasa we bought some Lux soap from the Friendship Store and took long, hot showers. I've never felt so clean in my life! To this day the smell of Lux, that pungent chemical perfume, takes me back to then: clean, safe and the proud owner of a sparkling ring.

Two months later, non-violent forms of protest broke out in Lhasa with demonstrations led by monks and nuns. At long last the Tibetans' struggle for independence became associated with demands for democracy and human rights. By 1989, Tibet was closed to foreigners, martial law had been declared and Chinese soldiers were positioned on rooftops. We'd got there just in time.

To be able to enjoy the adventures of each day in the knowledge that we had made this new commitment to each other was bliss. We sent postcards of Everest as engagement announcements, which much to everyone's amusement arrived home after us. Our wedding invitations were sealed with cut outs of Everest surrounded by a gold wedding ring, embossed in gold. On the day itself we served Everest-shaped chocolates with coffee ('*Qomolungma* chocolates', as written on the menu).

Memories of our four-day trip to Everest remain part of our marriage: they're part of our commitment to each other and the world.

3

The Axe Falls

On 16 September 1989 Andrew and I were married in the village of Aldbury, Hertfordshire. By this time, my parents had moved to the Isle of Harris, which I felt was too remote for the wedding and so I rang an old family friend, Margaret Kitson. In many ways, she was my surrogate granny. The retired schoolmistress of the old village school, she was in her eighties and had decided to learn Greek in order to read the Bible in Greek. She was a Christian with a youthful spirit, a zest for life and a fairytale cottage with low ceilings and creeping roses.

Margaret understood things in a way I've rarely encountered since. The most astute comment ever made about my relationship with Andrew came from her: she said that I prevent his feet from getting stuck to the ground and he stops me flying off altogether.

I'd always loved Aldbury. It's a picture-postcard English village with a village green, stocks and a duck pond. We were married in the Saint John the Baptist church. A local lady called Sue did the flowers and followed my then-unfashionable request for a trailing bouquet and crowns of flowers, the inspiration being *A Midsummer Night's Dream*. Mum and Dad had purchased my dress from Jenners, the then-independent equivalent of Harrods in Edinburgh. I made the veil, embroidered with seed pearls, which was attached to the crown of ivy and roses in my hair. My bridesmaids wore green – I'd made their dresses, too. Two of the girls hadn't been available for fittings and the dresses unfortunately gaped at the neckline so tissues were employed as stuffing. These came in handy when my grandmother had a nosebleed during the ceremony and hankies were produced from some rather unlikely places.

Our big day was everything we had hoped for: the sun came out and the setting was perfect, surrounded by family and friends. During the romantic carriage drive to the reception, Andrew and I remembered Everest and all it meant to us. The evening rang with the sounds of a ceilidh band, complete with caller, that I had managed to source. This type of dancing came as something of a surprise to our guests who were expecting the more predictable cheesy DJ and a few eighties' hits but everyone danced the night away.

In his wedding speech, Andrew talked of our shared challenge of reaching Everest and how important it was to us. We spent our honeymoon in Venice. Not that I realised it before we left – the trip was to be a surprise for me. All I knew was that we nearly missed our ferry: that morning over a leisurely breakfast Andrew suddenly remembered our passports were with his best man, who was rowing on the Thames. A worried phone call (still no mobile phones) brought the news that Adam was too hung-over to row. Instead he met us at a service station en route to hand over the passports. Phew!

With balloons and decorations flapping from the car, we arrived at the ferry terminal and were motioned on across an empty boarding area. Talk about last minute! We stayed one night in a small village in France and then another on the banks of Lake Geneva in a small, eccentric Swiss guesthouse; I still didn't know where we were headed. Eventually, we ended up in a sleepy little village called Chioggia over the bay from Venice, in a fisherman's tavern, and were wonderfully spoiled by the locals. We then moved on to Sienna, Giglio (a lovely island) and Florence.

Marriage suited us. Andrew and I are both children of strong marriages. My parents (Robin and John) met when they were teenagers and despite their differences have sustained a commitment that's still going strong; my in-laws' marriage I often imagine as a rock in stormy seas.

After the excitement of the wedding and all the travelling the return to reality came as a jolt. That autumn Andrew bought a new suit, had a haircut and started work as a surveyor looking after investment property portfolios in London. The job was interesting and meant that he could follow his dream of working in the City. After working eight weekends in a row at the Hospice, however, I was tired of shifts. No stranger to change, I applied and got onto a health-visiting course. This included practical and theory tuition in affiliation with a

GP's surgery in Lewisham, which was around the corner from where we were living in Catford (otherwise known as Forest Hill). It started as soon as we got back from our honeymoon. In fact, I missed the first week of the course.

By the time I was five, I'd lived in four different houses. Since I've been married to Andrew (21 years as I write this), I've lived in just three: I like the permanence of home, I like feeling settled. Our first flat was a two-bedroom conversion in a large Victorian house in Catford with high ceilings and a mantelpiece. A little bit of back garden was accessible through the front door and down the side alley. We completed at the height of the property boom and were seriously hit by negative equity but it was all ours. I purchased oddments of carpet and some second-hand blue velvet curtains and filled the window boxes with peonies, geraniums, trailing lobelia, fuchsias and marigolds.

On Christmas Eve we bought a Christmas tree that I decorated with red bows and white fairy lights. Andrew sat down. I sat on his lap and immediately fell fast asleep.

'We need a dog.'

It was Saturday morning. We were drinking tea and deciding whether to do the South Downs or more decorating. The best thing about weekends in London was being able to head out to the country or go into town to visit the museums and the theatre.

'I agree,' said Andrew.

We had reached the dog-owning stage of our lives. Both of us were dog lovers. Growing up as an only child, I'd always been grateful for their company. For my sixth birthday, Mum and Dad gave me Sandie, a gun-shy Gun Dog, who proved to be a great companion and partial to crisps. I was eating a packet of crisps when we went to get her. Unsurprisingly, she came to sit at my feet and obviously I thought, *she knows I'm her owner and that she's mine. What a clever girl!* She also loved hill walking as much as the rest of the family.

Sandie's way of expressing her displeasure at being left at home was to collect all the shoes in the house and leave them in a pile, mercifully undamaged, in the middle of the living room. She also disgraced herself almost immediately by eating the gingerbread house that Mum had baked for my birthday. Six months later she made a foray into the Christmas cake. We soon learnt about Labradors and food!

When I was 13 years old, Mum found a stray outside my school. We took the dog to the police pound but in the ensuing conversation with the on-duty policeman decided to keep him. Mum wasn't normally spontaneous but something about Shep made us fall in love with him. All black, he was possibly a Greyhound/Labrador mix, desperately thin and scared out of his wits; he had scabby paws, burns down one side and his ear had clearly been cut with scissors. The vet reckoned he had walked for miles. He might have been an unwanted Christmas present, living rough until he showed up outside school. Once we'd taken him home, he slept for three days and ate everything we put in front of him. He was so malnourished the vet warned that he could die if he wasn't carefully and gradually introduced to food.

The Axe Falls

Shep was a real rascal. Dad was convinced that had he been human he'd have worn a trilby and had a fag hanging from his mouth! He was also the most accident prone dog you could ever hope to meet: he caught his eye on the hook of the seat belt and ate a kilo of walnuts, which meant that he had to drink pints of liquid paraffin to get things moving. Mum reckons the South Downs haven't recovered from the mounds he deposited there – he had serious bellyache for weeks!

Shep and Sandie became firm friends. This was surprising given Sandie loathed every dog she met. In retrospect, it was good old-fashioned respect for his elders on Shep's part. The only exception to the rule was the single floor cushion that both dogs liked. If Shep happened to be on it, Sandie would charge to the front door, barking. This would lead to Shep getting up to investigate what all the noise was about. In a flash, Sandie would sneak over to take up residency on the coveted cushion.

Sandie died aged 14. By then, I was living away from home but I was devastated, as were my parents. Shep also went through a long period of mourning: he moped around the house, lost his appetite and generally looked glum.

Now that Andrew and I were committed to the search for a dog, autumn weekends were spent contacting local rescue charities. If you've ever been to a rescue centre or homing charity with the intention of getting a dog, you'll know exactly what I mean when I say it's an emotional rollercoaster: your heart races and the hairs on your arms stand on end. The chorus of lonely barks and whines, all those desperate faces, is like a magic formula – there's no way you'll be going home empty-handed.

A few weeks into the search one of the charities phoned to let us know that they had a suitable dog. He was living with a family who couldn't have him anymore. Jet was a year old and black, with grey eyes. He was part Black Labrador. Oh yes, and he had only three legs. Now you might think he wasn't an ideal dog, but again gut instinct told us he was the one. Jet was the first dog we met in our search and we knew he was right for us. He soon learned we loved him: he was our joker, he brought a lot of humour into our lives. We used to walk him in Beckenham Place Park or go for longer trips on the South Downs. His favourite game was playing tug. He could run so fast, he made heads turn. *My God, was that a three-legged dog?* You should have seen the expression on people's faces. Often we'd take him up to the Isle of Harris to visit my parents. They had a new dog called Lucy (Mum had given him to Dad for his birthday). Lucy was the most timid of the litter but with my parents' encouragement, she soon grew in confidence. She was an amazing dog, who knew the ways of the Island. Whenever we visited, Jet and Lucy played tug o' war with a long piece of rope that they had found washed up on the shore.

Life was settling into a routine that felt familiar and safe.

It was around this time that Andrew and I began volunteering for the Salvation Army Soup Kitchen. I can't remember who thought of it first but we ended up joining the team together. In the early nineties homelessness in London had become a huge problem and prejudice against the homeless was rife. As we soon learnt, there were lots of different types of homeless people: there were those who lived in cardboard boxes, with dreadlocks and dead eyes; others were confused and mentally ill, with all their worldly belongings stashed in a shopping trolley or single carrier bag. There were also army veterans of all ages and businessmen who had lost everything, declared themselves bankrupt and walked away unable to face the shame. The Colonel was an army veteran who lived under the South Bank and knew an underground route into Covent Garden Theatre, where you could get the best standing positions for the proms. We also spent ages listening to a man whose wife and daughter had both died – he didn't want to go on without them.

On Friday nights we would go and pick up the van from the Salvation Army Hall in Peckham and make a tour of the city's homeless spots. London's bright lights were dimmer, less jewel-like, from the vantage point of a van filled with free food for the disadvantaged. We did the South Bank, Waterloo, Regent Street and the Embankment giving out sandwiches donated by Marks & Spencer; there were urns of tea and coffee plus homemade soup prepared earlier by volunteers. To this day I can summon the smell of soup and tea and petrol, and with it memories of long nights dispensing help and hearing stories from people who I grew genuinely fond of. We only felt scared a couple of times. Once we were in the Bull Ring (a notorious underground area): on Andrew's barked instructions, we all leapt into the van whereupon people jumped on the roof and kicked it. Andrew got us all out safely and that, thankfully, was the exception rather than the rule.

We gave out blankets and clothes before driving home, shattered, at 3am just before the dawn chorus. But I genuinely loved the work and admired people's dignity: we would open the van doors to a crowd of people, all of whom had preferences.

'I don't like ham. Do you have any cheese and pickle?'

I had infinite respect for the way in which they asserted their right to choose, even if it was for mayonnaise rather than mustard.

To be perfectly honest, I'd say my altruism partly stems from a selfish interest in people; I'm interested in society's marginalised groups. Later, when I worked with the Kurdish refugees who had fled after the first Gulf War and then the gypsies in Kent (where I set up a three-year healthcare project), I began to think about the implications for us all of those who society rejects. What does it say about us?

By now, in the summer of 1990, I was coming to the end of my health-visitors' course. As part of my studies, I travelled to an alternative practice down in Wiltshire, where I had a two-week country placement. Wiltshire meant an escape from London's concrete jungle and the chance to stay with our wonderful friends, Ruth and Jack. It was a blissfully hot summer; the hedgerows were full of foxgloves and apple blossom scent filled the air. I loved driving along the country lanes where sunlight flashed through the woods. Ruth and Jack lived in a cottage with an enormous garden and every day after work Jack would hand me a glass of chilled white wine made from his own grapes. Glass in hand, I would go and lie down on the lawn … and nod off! Ruth had been left severely disabled by polio and their marriage was something Andrew and I always admired and gained strength from over the years.

Fatigue had plagued me for most of that year, as had my left eye. My vision was impaired by what looked like a hair or cobweb floating in front of it but I put this down to studying too hard. When my placement came to an end, I was sorry to say goodbye to Jack and Ruth. I drove back up to the stench and noise of London to resume work.

But I didn't feel well.

I went to see my GP with chronic backache and a problem peeing (I assumed it was a urinary infection). The GP prescribed antibiotics and sent off a specimen. The following Monday, 18 June (the day before my birthday), I woke to no feeling at all from the waist down on my right-hand side (I remember thinking, *I must have cramp – I should eat some salt and I mustn't be late for work*). I got up and discovered that I could walk but I had no feeling. As usual, I jogged round the park with Jet before driving along the road to work. I didn't want to worry anyone at work with my numb leg, so I didn't say anything about it.

Mid-morning, I fell down the stairs. I couldn't feel my foot – I couldn't tell whether I'd put it down on the stair or not. I mentioned the problem to my supervisor, who immediately whisked me off to see my GP, who happened to be in the same building.

'What do you mean, by no feeling?' he asked.

I leant over his desk and picked up a safety pin.

'This is what I mean ...'

I proceeded to stick the pin in my leg.

The GP rang a friend and registrar at the National Hospital for Nervous Diseases to make an appointment for me to go and see him later that week on the Thursday. On my birthday (19 June), Andrew drove us to Down House in Kent, where Charles Darwin had lived and worked for 40 years. It was where he devised his Theory of Evolution and wrote *On the Origin of Species*. According to the guide when Darwin published his work in 1859 the experience was akin to 'confessing a murder', which gives some indication of its impact. The impression you take away from the house is of a playful man, who loved digging for worms and ragging with his children. My admiration for him grew.

Andrew and I had dinner in a pub but neither of us knew what to say. We went for a walk in the woods. Drugged by the scent of wild garlic and bluebells, we walked hand-in-hand in silence. Despite the sunshine, I felt bitterly cold and didn't take my coat off all day.

On my return to hospital I was immediately admitted upstairs for more tests. I was hooked up to IV steroids to prevent inflammation and further damage to the nerves. My face blew up and I had tomato-red cheeks but there was worse to come in the form of a myelogram, which is when dye is injected into the spine to show up the spinal nerves and spinal canal. I had a major reaction to the dye, which made me more ill than I already was.

Tired and now in immense pain as if suffering from chemically induced meningitis, I lay in the hot, over-crowded ward with a splitting headache. It hurt to breathe and I couldn't pee so I had to have a catheter. With a cloth over my eyes and my head ready to explode, I lay there as the nurses' hand-washing routine ground into my consciousness. It was in the days before disinfectant hand gel and every few minutes one of them would walk over to the sink beside my bed, turn on the squeaking tap, wash her hands and pull out a paper towel. Rustle, rustle … I'd then hear the click as she stamped on the bin and the thud of paper as the screwed-up towel landed inside. During this time, Andrew would come and go; he was mixing caring for me, his full-time work and dashing back home to look after Jet, traversing London all the time.

Mum came to visit and gave me two new nightdresses. One was crisp Broderie Anglaise, the other a comfy long T-shirt. She also brought books and magazines, sitting beside me to read. Company was what I needed as much as anything else.

Towards the end of my week on the ward, on one particularly hot afternoon I sensed someone sitting on the bed. I can't emphasise enough how much I felt this presence. It was before the drugs took effect and I couldn't open my eyes because of the pain; I remember a gorgeous smell of gardenias, as if a nurse wearing perfume was sitting right beside me. I must have said something.

'Who are you talking to?' asked the on-duty nurse.

'The nurse sitting on my bed,' I replied.

'There's no one here apart from me and I haven't sat on your bed,' she told me.

For me, this was proof of my faith and it brought immense comfort.

After seven days of waiting and six sleepless nights spent tossing and turning, I woke to learn that I would be seeing the consultant on that morning's ward round (Andrew was at work and couldn't be there with me).

I sat up in my bed. It was far too early, of course – you never know when they will arrive nor from which end of the ward they start. Up until then I had only dealt with the Registrar. This time I was to meet my consultant. As usual the entourage arrived: the line-up included the Charge Nurse (why do they always look so deferential and play up to the pomposity of consultants?), multiple medical students, house officers and the Registrar. The beds were so close together due to overcrowding that you could put your hand out and hold the hand of a fellow patient in a neighbouring bed. Even with the flimsy curtains closed, privacy was impossible.

I heard the Registrar tell the lady next door they were moving her to a hospice. She had an inoperable brain tumour, which put things into perspective.

Doing my best to ignore the banging in my head and the nausea, I tried to sit upright.

'Good morning,' said the Registrar. 'Sally, do you mind if my medical student here does a brief examination?'

'No,' I insisted. 'That's fine.'

First, he got the student to look at me and asked me not to give any clues as to my condition. The student discovered the numbness ran in a spiral pattern down my back. Following this, the consultant then told the student, 'That's how you can assess how truthful a patient is being – they don't know about the spiral effect.'

Great. Someone believes me, I thought.

Then the consultant – a portly, elderly gentleman in a bow tie and half-moon glasses – stepped forward. They all tried to crowd round him but there wasn't enough room and so a couple of hapless students (the type who get into med school because they're brilliant but don't realise patients are people) tried to squeeze in around the curtain, leaving it gaping to the world.

I hadn't realised I was being examined by the consultant until I suddenly found that he was addressing me.

'... So, having ruled out various other diseases, sarcoidosis and tumours, what we're looking at is Multiple Sclerosis, hopefully of the relapse-remitting kind.'

I looked up to a sea of faces.

'We will discharge you for now but you will have a recall for an MRI scan that will give us final confirmation and see if you have had any other attacks in the past.'

That was it.

As a nurse I had half-expected the diagnosis yet it still came as a shock: the world slowed down. I wanted to ask a million questions but the consultant and doctors had already swept past and were onto the next bed. No information was given; there was no opportunity for discussion.

What are the implications? I silently screamed.

It was a harsh lesson and a taste of things to come. MS is an incurable disease: the medics don't want to spend time discussing it with you. What's there to talk about?

I was left alone and I can honestly say I've never felt so alone as I did then.

Everything I'd dreamt about – the travelling, excitement, the future together we had planned – ground to a halt. No dreaming of Shangri-La. Instead I faced a life stuck … with what? As I packed and prepared to leave the ward with Andrew, who had by now arrived, the nurses came up and gave me hugs. One stopped herself mid-sentence: 'I hope you'll get bet – … I hope things work out well for you.'

We drove home in silence. Everything looked so different: the colours were brighter. After a week's internment in a grey hospital I had a new vision of life, its preciousness and brutality. I couldn't halt the flood of anxieties. *What if the MS hits my eyes and I can't see or it affects my arms and I can't hold a pen? Will I ever be able to climb another mountain again or ride a horse?*

Horse riding was something I'd learned in Scotland while studying to become a nurse. I'd drive over to the stables and go cantering across the open fields; I'd come to love the sound of hooves drumming on the ground, the roar of the horses' breath.

There were a million unanswered questions, each one scarier than the last. I was so terrified and confused. Yet, believe it or not, amid the fear and uncertainty was a feeling of relief and with it a sort of calm: the past two years had a reason. Those mysterious symptoms weren't laziness or my going mad – they were real, *very* real.

As a nurse I was able to understand the physiology of the disease but I made the choice not to inform myself too much. The more I knew, the worse my anxiety would be over what to expect. The strangely reassuring news was that I had suffered other attacks, with scarring in my cerebellum (a region of the brain), which explained the dizziness and exhaustion. I could have had it for some time and not known until it felled me.

I had an image of myself, running and climbing, partying and laughing while the black net of MS ensnared me – and finally tripped me up. My thoughts turned to Andrew and his pain when he heard the diagnosis, his utter devastation, and I knew that I would have to be strong for us both. The uncertainty of what lay ahead, the sense of imminent loss, was extremely hard.

It was also very hard for Andrew.

Andrew is a very centred person; he never complains. I kept apologising: *I'm so sorry, I'm so sorry. If you'd known about this, you wouldn't have married me.*

'There aren't "what-ifs" in marriage,' he told me. 'I married *you* and that includes in sickness and in health – no one knows what that involves.'

I felt horribly guilty but Andrew was tremendous: he got me through it all by being so calm and loving. Later on he confessed he hadn't known what to do. At lunch-times when I was back at the hospital having more tests, he would find a quiet church somewhere in the city to pray. Our best man, a lovely man called Adam who used to work nearby, came to see me.

'Can you look after Andrew?' I asked. 'It's harder for him than it is for me – he's the one watching the illness.'

Back at home my fear wasn't helped by the bombardment of contradictory advice. My GP advised lots of exercise and less sleep. Meanwhile, the MS Society sent more leaflets with news of handrails and catheters, which in retrospect was entirely unnecessary. More useful would have been day-to-day guidelines such as to be careful when taking a bath. I ran a bath and got in, scalding myself, because I couldn't feel the temperature. The things I had always taken for granted had now vanished: my entire life would need to be reassessed.

I called my friend – a doctor, who was also one of my bridesmaids – to tell her that I'd been diagnosed with MS. She said her boyfriend had died paragliding the previous week; I felt guilty for feeling self-pity. I then heard that one of my other friends who was also training to become a health visitor had been diagnosed with Stage 3 ovarian cancer and another fellow student was to have a lung/heart transplant as her cystic fibrosis had worsened.

So, I was the lucky one.

The good news was that the summer of 1990 was a great one for lying on the sofa. Martina Navratilova won her ninth Wimbledon and Gazza wept as England was knocked out in the World Cup semi-finals by Germany. I had the windows open and Jet (my therapy pet) beside me, keeping me company. During this time, I slept a lot. Trying to adjust to the constant pain and the strange sensation similar to having cotton wool wrapped around my legs brought a mire of emotions and confusion. What I knew was that MS doesn't get better – in fact, it just gets worse as the condition is incurable – but I didn't have a clue what to do.

Just then I was happy to be home with Jet.

For ages I'd had my eye on the empty greenhouse next door. After the MS attack our neighbour, a kindly old gent, offered me the use of it. He even created a little gate in the fence to make it easier for me to enter. Now I grew thousands of tomatoes – we had to buy a freezer to store them all. I also cultivated flowers from seeds in a desire to nurture and feel closer to nature.

In the October my Aunt Pat and Uncle Andy arranged for us to rent Pat's parents' apartment in the Canary Islands and also to borrow their car. I fell and ripped my leg to shreds on the volcanic rocks but it didn't hurt because I still had no feeling.

So that was OK then, I remember thinking. After all, there was no point in crying. Retaining a sense of humour was crucial and was to bolster me in my darkest hours.

4

Bumpy Road

As soon as I was able to resume work, I began a new job as a health visitor in Lewisham. I was perfectly candid about my MS with the staff – I didn't hide my condition from anyone. Besides, I'd had to delay the probation period as I was still in hospital when I was due to start. Luckily, I'd almost made a full recovery as far as walking was concerned. I still had the strange numbness in my leg and the lower right side of my back but at least I wasn't on medication and so I was able to start enjoying life again despite the curveball thrown at me.

As part of a primary healthcare team, it was my job to assess the needs of the individual, the family and the wider community. This involved house visits on a number of different estates. And OK, there was abuse, misery and poverty but also an amazing sense of community: the Jamaicans especially were brilliant. This was when I discovered Jamaican food: I did battle with the scales on an emperor fish and overdid jerk paste on the chops. We attended a fantastic Nigerian christening and a Chinese wedding – I was steeped in previously alien cultures. I was glad to be able to say 'hello' in Cantonese and know if they were being rude to me – which quite often they were.

The area was full of high-rise flats and appallingly deprived estates with broken windows and graffiti. Hallways and lifts (when they worked) stank of stale urine. I had to walk over syringes and used condoms to get up 12 flights because the lifts weren't working ... again. Sometimes the flats themselves were just as bad. Other times I would knock, the door would open and I'd find myself in a beautifully kept home. However, I did get a shock when visiting a family to discuss infection control (their daughter had just been diagnosed with lymphoma). Sitting on the settee, I felt and then spotted a large snake sliding along the back of the settee.

'Don't worry about the boa,' said the dad. 'She's harmless.'

It was around this time that Anne Diamond's cot death campaign was gathering momentum, with lots of TV and newspaper coverage. There was endless talk of positioning babies and low birth-weights. But the mums that I saw – Nigerian, Chinese, Jamaican, and Kurdish refugees – didn't have cots: they were busy trying to survive. What's more, they slept with their babies, often until they were five years old.

One day a mum covered in tattoos came to see me.

'Can you come and see my son?' she asked. 'I'm worried about his language.'

Two days later, as arranged, I went to their flat. I rang the door. It opened and a little boy looked up.

'Who the fuck are you?'

The mum quickly came to the door (his father was in prison for GBH).

'Well,' I observed. 'He doesn't seem to have any language problems.'

'Yes, he does,' she insisted. 'And I don't know where the fuck he gets it from!'

Trying to assess the effectiveness of your work as a health visitor can be difficult. There are only so many follow-up visits you can make but I knew I had secured the trust of the women on the estate when one of them introduced me by saying, 'This is Sally. You can't get her to lie for you, but she won't dob you in.'

In other words, I wouldn't report them to Benefits or Housing. I would, however, report to Social Services if I had any concerns about their kids. There were so many life-or-death situations. Children on the Child Protection Register were relatively safe; they had routine visits. It was the 'grey areas' – the kids who weren't on the Register – where there was no proof of abuse that you had to worry about. They were the cases that kept you up at night. With nearly 300 families on my caseload, what could I do?

Sometimes my efforts were in vain. I once saw a young Latin-American woman whose husband was abusing her; it was a clear case of domestic violence. She was hiding her bruises and despite gentle probing would never admit it to me. It was also difficult to get her alone as she spoke very little English. Then one day she came into the health-care centre, crying. Moments later her husband charged in, wielding a kitchen knife: the three of us (and their baby) were in my office. Outside, a crowd of women and babies were in the waiting room. I handed the baby over to a nurse, who quickly vacated the room. Eventually I talked the husband down and listened to what he had to say, that he just wanted his baby. Following this, I promptly got on the phone to try and secure the wife a place in the Latin-American women's refuge but it was all the way up in north London. The husband agreed to leave but to come back and see me the next day. Meanwhile, the woman left with the police and her baby, but the police wouldn't take her to the refuge: they would only put her on the Tube so I gave her the money for the fare. The next thing I heard, she had taken her baby and gone back to her husband.

Throughout this time, my sanity was Jet. Before and after work, I would take him for long walks, relishing the green after a day in the grime. We were now in the spring of 1991. Tuesday morning. As usual, I took Jet for a walk before work at Beckenham Place Park, which backed onto some big estates. This was before the craze for Staffordshire Bull Terriers but there were a lot of other vicious dogs around. One moment Jet was sniffing a bush, the next thing he was being attacked by a large Alsatian – he tried to run away but it was hopeless. I shouted at the owner to control her dog and she casually called him. The Alsatian released Jet and followed his owner out of the park, leaving me to rush over and pick up my own dog. Panting, he was visibly in pain. I drove him to the vet. An hour later, my worst fears were realised: the vet informed me that the knee-joint of Jet's one and only back leg had been fatally damaged.

'I'm very sorry,' he said. 'He only had three legs to start with. You're going to have to put him down.'

Heart-broken, I broke down and sobbed. The pain was physical: my body ached with the loss of my best friend. Some lovely friends of ours went to the house and removed all of Jet's things before I got home so that we didn't have to deal with the trauma of seeing them. Throughout my diagnosis, subsequent recuperation and the first few months of learning to live with MS, Jet had been my rock.

How do you learn to live with fear? I'm still looking for the answer to that one.

All I knew was that the mornings were now filled with dread as I woke to discover which bit of my body was, or wasn't, working. Andrew and I had in a sense been ignoring the MS so that it wouldn't become central to our lives. Instead I used to whisper my fears to Jet as a way of sharing the sadness; I'd tell him how much pain I suffered over my altered body image (I'd prided myself on my strength). He would listen patiently as I wept over lost opportunities and wagged his tail when I told him how glad I was that Andrew had travelled, had really lived and been so active before I was struck down by the disease.

Some people in our church were of the view that I should pray for a healing yet my feeling was that if I was to be healed then it would happen. Jet's bravery was an inspiration: I only had to watch him bound across the park with his determined three-legged run to feel better about everything. He could always bring a smile to my face but now he was gone.

Bumpy Road

It would be another 20 years until I had another dog and under very different circumstances – which says a lot about Jet.

To try and make up for the loss, Andrew and I plunged ourselves into work. That August we went camping in Czechoslovakia. We drove all the way there, which allowed us the freedom to go where and when we wanted on our adventure. It was 1991 and only two years after the Berlin Wall had come down; everything was insanely cheap. The further East we went, the more deprivation we witnessed: shops became emptier and the stunning scenery was unexpectedly interrupted by a huge toxic lake or mine. Everywhere we went we encountered friendly, hospitable people and simple, but well maintained campsites. Camping, it seemed, was a Czech national pastime. We visited Wenceslas Square in Prague, where in 1969 a freedom fighter set himself alight. I remember my dad talking about him and really we went there on his behalf. Towards the end of our trip everyone started to look worried and warned us to stay close to the border. On our return, we read in an English newspaper that Mikhail Gorbachev had stood on the tanks in Red Square. The Czechs were concerned that the Russians were once more about to invade.

Our trip to Czechoslovakia proved more fruitful than expected. Nine months later, on 14 May 1992, my beautiful, dark-haired son was born in Lewisham Hospital. In the early days after my diagnosis the doctors stressed the risks of pregnancy and how it could trigger a relapse of the MS but it was a risk I was prepared to take. At the time they also told me that MS wasn't genetic, although now of course there is evidence of a significantly higher chance of diagnosis if another family member is a sufferer. They also believe there is a female-to-female connection given the sex has a higher predisposition to the disease. This risk is one for which I feel tremendous guilt; I wouldn't wish MS on anyone – it's terrible but no one has found a gene for it.

There was no mistaking whose child he was: here was a mini-Andrew, who looked very similar to my husband's maternal grandfather, whose giggle I can still hear. We christened him Peter after the patron saint of Czechoslovakia.

So now I was a mother, who also happened to have MS.

It wasn't an easy birth – I had a long labour, an epidural, episiotomy ... the works. Nor were my three days in the hospital all that comfortable. At the time breastfeeding was frowned upon: clever mums bottle-fed their babies. I'll never forget the first long night of motherhood (who can?) as I struggled to get to grips with breastfeeding. How could I get Peter to latch on, suck, burp, latch on, suck ... oh and then change him? He screamed and screamed.

'What's wrong with that baby?' I overheard one of the nurses complain to her colleague.

'It's a breast-feeder,' said the other.

They put a notice on the cot: *Do not bottlefeed this baby.* For three long days, I couldn't move because of my stitches. At some point, I asked a passing nurse, 'Can you take my baby?'

'No, it's a breast-feeder. We can't put him in the nursery,' came the reply.

As a nurse, I found the attitude of the nurses indefensible: I needed a gentle, comforting word. As for the family planning nurse, she didn't stay long! Three months later, I went back in to have a general anaesthetic and my cut re-sutured.

And so life as a mother began.

Back in Catford I would push Peter through the streets in his buggy. Later, Andrew came home from work, changed out of his suit and I handed the baby over to him. We were both drowning with exhaustion from having an unsettled child; also Andrew was working very long hours. I was still madly in love with Andrew just craving time for myself and a little sleep.

How I wept over those Hallmark cards sent by kind friends with their cloying messages for happy, coping mums, not Mums like me. I remember feeling alone and very resentful: part of it, I think, was missing work and in retrospect, the effects of the MS (not that there was any time to pay attention to it back then). Not only was I a new mum, but I had chronic fatigue too and my soul was yearning for green. Though I liked London life, I missed the countryside. When Peter was six months old, I went back to work part-time but with the same caseload.

We had a big plum tree in the garden at Catford: our little patch of green in London. For Peter's first birthday we bought him a swing that we hung under it. Around the same time, I applied for – and landed – a part-time job setting up and running a healthcare project for gypsies with a district nurse in Maidstone, Kent. Although the journey was nearly an hour long, I rejoiced in getting us both out into the countryside surroundings. As I looked back from the hill where the nursery was located, I could see the Canary Wharf Tower semi-masked by yellow, polluted haze. Andrew used to cycle to work into the thick of it. In vain, I begged him to wear a mask.

Every time we drove up to Scotland, we would return with a growing sense of gloom. As soon as we hit the old M1 and the build-up of concrete and looked at London again, I'd feel a pit of dread in my stomach. Then I'd start to cry. My longing for green had been there ever since I started work at Guy's; it was the same sense of claustrophobia that made me go out and buy big bunches of daffodils from the local flower-seller and arrange them in vases all round the flat.

One day, on the way back from work in Maidstone I spotted a derelict property in Beckenham. It was a Victorian end-of-terrace with bow windows, a big garden and a lime tree in the front. I told Andrew to go and take a look. The next day he peered over the fence. We rang the estate agent and put in an offer without even going inside. It turned out to have sixties' mustard nylon carpets and peeling wallpaper; also the loveliest veranda at the back, glass-roofed and covered in vines. Depending on your point of view, this was a homeowner's dream (or nightmare). Luckily, the vendors were very understanding and allowed us to start work before completion: the whole house had to be rewired and have gas and central heating installed.

My family means everything to me. It's full of snapshots, moments entirely unplanned and often it's the small ones that stand out most.

Here's one: Peter and I are sitting on the steps outside the new house on a dark morning. I'm on my way to work but we're waiting for the gasman to show up. We're having a 'Paddington Bear' breakfast: eating Marmalade sandwiches out of a suitcase (lunchbox). I'm drinking tea from the flask. Peter decides to go off exploring with his Thomas the Tank Engine torch. He opens the door to enter the house and falls into a hole in the floor. Thankfully, he isn't hurt – just a couple of scratches – but the expression of surprise and relief on his face as I yank him out makes my heart melt.

He's my little soldier. Still is.

At last we moved in. Even though the house was chaos, I was so much happier. What's more, we managed to rent out the Catford flat to avoid negative equity. We put Peter's wellies by the back door: at the age of two and three-quarters he could open the back door, put on his wellies and wander off into the walled garden.

Peter was lucky to be alive, or rather I was lucky to have him alive. Just before he was two we'd had a nasty scare that still resonated for all the usual parental reasons: the 'what-ifs' and the 'if-onlys'. Peter was an allergic child.

As a baby he'd suffered severe eczema and so I switched his milk to soya. One afternoon, we'd gone along to our local Turkish delicatessen to pick up a few things for supper and a snack for Peter. I bought him a carton of apple juice and some halva, which he'd never tried before: as sesame seeds are full of calçium, I thought it would be a fantastic healthy snack. It looked so delicious lying beside the counter in the tray that I couldn't resist.

Peter was in his buggy. I paid the man, gave my son a tiny piece of halva to suck on and left the shop. He began making a choking sound as if something was stuck in his throat and so I leant over the top of the buggy and gave him his juice.

'Take a sip, love,' I said.

He started to scream. I rushed round to find him covered from head to toe in hives; it looked like a nettle rash. Thanks to my professional training, I recognised it at once as anaphylactic shock. The next sequence of events seemed to last forever; it was life in slow motion. I ran down the street to the cab firm with no money in my purse and told the driver: 'I've got to get my son to the hospital *now*!'

While we were driving, Peter stopped breathing. I started to resuscitate him. The driver, a Jamaican man, kept his hand on the horn. We went through red lights, down side streets and into the hospital emergency drop-off. I picked up Peter, ran into hospital and like a miracle, found a registrar standing there and handed him Peter.

'He's in respiratory arrest. I think it's an anaphylactic shock,' I said.

Bumpy Road

I had to sign a consent form for a tracheostomy. Peter was awake but needed IV antihistamine. They checked his oxygen levels. Then the Sister asked, 'Where's his dad?'

Everything is OK … Oh no, they want his dad! Things aren't OK.

That day, Andrew was working in the centre of London. I rang him and he called someone else from our church to ask, 'Can you go and support Sally while I make my way there.' By the time he had borrowed a car to get there, Peter was out of the resuscitation area: he was tomato-red from head to toe and couldn't swallow because his throat was so swollen. He was placed in a ward in a cot and I was terrified to let him out of my sight. But then the curate from our church appeared: he stayed with Peter while I got something to eat (I wanted to spend the night on the paediatric ward). Back then there were no beds for parents and so after sending Andrew home to sleep (he had work in the morning), I spent the night sitting beside the cot.

The next day, as Peter was discharged with adrenalin and syringes, we were given our lives back. It was a terrifying way to find out that halva contains sesame and peanut oil and Peter is allergic to both.

I was newly pregnant at the time, with the baby due the following February: we had been sure that we wanted a sibling for Peter. Again, I was lucky and my health was excellent during the pregnancy apart from a severe pelvic muscle pain that made walking difficult but I did it. Mums do, don't they?

*   *   *

It was courtesy of a gypsy that I found out that I was carrying a girl. Just before Peter's first birthday I spotted an advert in the *Nursing Times* for a gypsy project in Kent:

> *Wanted: A Health Visitor to join a district nurse already in post to care for the travelling population of Maidstone district.*

Or words to that effect. It was such a tiny advert. When I imagined rural Kent, my mind filled with fruit farms, trees and fields. I'd had enough of the concrete jungle. *Great, it's a job I can do in wellies!* was my first reaction; my second thought was that establishing trust was key to this particular role and from the experience of working in Lewisham I knew this to be one of my strengths. Kent Family Health Services Authority wanted to establish outreach primary care services for traveller families in mid-Kent. Put simply, someone had carried out a study and subsequently realised the infant mortality rate in their community was way too high: something needed to be done.

Elvira was the clan's matriarch. Traditionally, the matriarch of a site is responsible for sanctioning relations between healthcare workers and the gypsies. An amazing woman with waist-length, jet-black hair, she had a mother who lived with them whom I saw rarely but who seemed ancient as the woods. They lived in a tolerated site (illegal but hidden away, where no one would move them on) in the middle of some woods, up a dirt track. In the clearing

were six mobile homes and one or two temporary caravans. Elvira's own home was spotless: it was crowded
with precious nick-nacks and china, lace curtains and a
gorgeous wood-burning stove (a temporary caravan was
next door for the men to sit in and 'mess up' after work).
She had a pet jackdaw who would sit on the open door
and come if called.

One day, after visiting, I tripped slightly going down
the steps.

'Careful,' she warned. 'Take care of your little girl in
there!'

Stunned, I stopped in my tracks.

'Sorry, I try not to do that,' she said, looking
embarrassed.

I was exactly three weeks and two days pregnant with
Clara but I had no idea at the time that I was carrying my
daughter. Incredible!

Three weeks before Clara was born, we moved into
our new home in Beckenham. I had wanted a home-birth
but was deemed too high-risk because of my MS. Luckily
I'd already made friends with Diane, a senior midwife at
Maidstone Hospital: a wonderful woman and a midwife
in the best sense of the word. Diane believed in the benefits of water births and championed their effectiveness in
pain management and the gravitational pull that enables
the pelvis to open and the baby to slip out – and she was
right.

On 19 February 1995, Clara shot out like a slippery
fish and was placed on my chest. The difference between
the births of my two children couldn't have been more

dramatic. After the skin tears and cutting I'd had to endure with Peter, the experience of an underwater birth was bliss and so empowering. For the majority of the time Andrew and I were left alone to enjoy the experience of birth in a way I'd previously thought unimaginable. Afterwards, as Clara was being checked, weighed, and swaddled, I had the best tea and toast known to womankind. Ah, the delights of NHS hospitality!

I spent the night on the ward. The next day Diane carried Clara out of the hospital in her car seat (it was the midwife's job, that was the rule). Peter came running up and tried to kick her in the shins.

'Leave my baby sister alone!' he shouted.

I couldn't help but feel proud.

Clara was happiest lying in her pram, looking up at the hanging vines. Our world was contained within that walled garden: we were oblivious to the racket outside – the busy main road, shoppers, cars and nightclub queues on Friday nights. Indoors, we installed double-glazing. Andrew built a tree-boat (as opposed to a tree-house) in two trees at the end of the garden so that Peter could sail to Timbuctoo. I covered the end of his boat with curtains made from cheerful striped cotton strung from a wire. It wasn't long before Peter and his school-friend Simon discovered the best game in the world: shooting water pistols at unsuspecting passers-by on the pavement below.

And of course, we had the trains. From the tree-boat you could see the roof of the Beckenham Junction station. What more could a little boy want?

Bumpy Road

So why did I feel so blue? After the births of each of my children, I felt increasingly overwhelmed and with anxiety came depression. It wasn't so bad with Peter but I felt its grip tighten after the birth of Clara. Trying to unravel the symptoms of MS from possible signs of post-natal depression and the normal feelings of life-change associated with motherhood can be very difficult.

My reaction to the pressures of now having two kids was an urgent need for order: I was manic. By 8am, I'd have the kids washed and fed, the kitchen swept, the dish-washer on and would start calling people, while wondering, why aren't they being more chatty? I went to see the GP to talk about my feelings of inadequacy and frustration, my mania, and she diagnosed post-natal depression and suggested a course of anti-depressants.

Because of my MS I was allocated a community psychiatric nurse, who after two visits was signed off with stress and so that was that. I wasn't unduly alarmed. Lots of mums suffer PND, usually in response to fatigue and a sense of being overwhelmed; it heals over time. I refused the anti-depressants and battled the depression until it lifted, which it finally did.

Looking back, I don't think I allowed enough leeway for the MS, by which I mean that I didn't want my condition to impact on other peoples' attitudes towards me. Perhaps I was in denial, maybe I should have had more support – after all, MS exhaustion is the sort of exhaustion that sleep doesn't remedy. My exhaustion (made twenty times worse by the MS) in turn triggered feelings of guilt that I wasn't doing enough.

Driving the kids home one day, I fell asleep at the wheel. We were on a motorway. Thank God for the rumble strips at the side of the motorway, which woke me up! I parked up in the lane and took a deep breath, adrenalin coursing through my veins. If I'd known then what I know now, I'd have been able to say it's the MS, not me. Instead lodged in my head was a comment made by the GP after my first big bout of MS.

'You need to break this sleeping habit,' he told me. 'Pull yourself together.'

So I didn't put it down to MS – I assumed it was my failure as a mother.

In retrospect, I don't think the medical community could have helped: you have to be pretty bad to be entitled to respite care. Besides, I wanted to look after my kids and I wanted to work. I wanted it all. Why shouldn't I?

Just as I did with Peter, when Clara was six months old I put her in a nursery and went back to work. I had mixed emotions but there was also the relief of being able to sit down, plan my day and drink a hot cup of coffee. This, however, was undermined by anxiety over how the kids were faring and guilt that I myself should be caring for them. I always felt better after I'd collected them, seen how happy they were and I learned how active they had been during the day. Anyway, I was still with them well over 50 per cent of the time, I forced myself to remember.

5

Gypsy Life

My new job in Kent was wonderful. Although I didn't have any experience of working with travellers (or gypsies, as they prefer to be known), I had dealt with ethnic minority groups such as Kurds and Vietnamese. Gypsies were by then recognised as an ethnic minority and the project team in Kent was eager to identify the needs associated with different types of gypsy. They didn't want to be called 'travellers' and therefore tarred with the same brush as the New Age and the Irish.

I quickly discovered that there are lots of different groups of gypsy and each one has its own approach to medical care. There were the New Age travellers who lived in converted buses. I met one lot who lived in tree-houses, like something out of Enid Blyton's *The Faraway Tree*, with the branches disappearing into clouds (no sign of 'Moon-Face', 'Mr Watzisname' or 'Angry Pixie', however). These weren't eco-warriors but tree-dwellers. Thank goodness I could still climb ladders back then! There were the Irish, who travelled with the motorway works and produced tarmac drives on the side. I also interacted with settled Romanies and most elusive of all, Romanies on the move.

There were 15 gypsy encampments, in and around Maidstone; they tended to park up on brown field sites. Driving past, you'd see the typical disarray of caravans, old vans, kids and dogs. What impressed me most and dispelled all those myths was their strict observation of the rules of hygiene; they lived in immaculate caravans and were wonderful people. OK, there were rogues too, but the gypsy community was a microcosm of society at large: hard workers and layabouts.

According to tradition, I was always served tea in the cracked cup reserved for non-gypsies (they would never dream of using a cracked item). Also, I washed my hands in a separate bowl to the one used by the gypsies. I remember asking one very elusive group of girls (who would, however, give me a call when they were nearby) why they thought non-gypsies were dirty.

'Because you let your dogs sleep with you and eat in your house. And you wash your tea towels with your knickers.'

Great answer.

As a point of liaison between the gypsies and Maidstone Hospital, one of my first responsibilities was to admit a six-month-old baby with bronchiolitis (inflammation of the lungs), whose mum was just 15 years old. When a child from the gypsy community is in hospital, everyone comes to visit; before you know it, there are 40 visitors. Part of my job was to explain infection control. I had to persuade the immediate family to stay in the area so we could do follow-up care and ensure the baby's proper recovery. However, I then found out that the law had changed: gypsies could no longer park up for reasons of ill health or death.

Taking matters (OK, and the law) into my own hands, I persuaded the family to park up on a little triangle of land managed by Savills beside the motorway. Within 12 hours, they faced the threat of eviction. I drove over there and parked my car. I was wearing a flowery dress: the police came to move the gypsies on and assumed I was one of them. But I wasn't moving: instead I sat on the tow-bar of the caravan.

'There's a sick baby here who needs to see the community paediatric nurse,' I said.

'I could have you arrested for obstruction,' the policeman told me, hands on hips.

'Well, I could go to the papers and tell them that a health visitor was arrested while trying to care for a sick baby.'

'Oh!'

But I didn't win the argument: we did, however, gain a 24-hour reprieve. I drove ahead of the gypsies and showed them a little place where I knew they would be relatively safe. So, as well as working as a liaison with the hospital I was now expert in planning law and housing rights for gypsies and travellers. I knew all the hiding spaces: the gypsies used to follow me and I would lead them into the woods where they could pitch. Again, it goes back to my belief in social justice and a need to help those deprived of their rights. I sympathise with people whose views and lands are obstructed, sometimes even destroyed by travellers: I don't defend that sort of 'occupation' but I do defend the gypsy's right to a stable home environment.

You might say I became too involved but it wasn't sheer bloody-mindedness that compelled me to do what I could to make a difference: the welfare of children was at stake.

The day Elvira's mother passed away in the October of 1995 was a sad occasion for everyone. Buried with her were Romany traditions and customs that in my opinion would never return. My impression was that the community was mourning a way of life when she died. Traditionally, a gypsy body is cremated inside a caravan but this practice was illegal. However, it was customary to leave the body in the caravan and invite everyone to the wake; it is also a tradition to keep a fire alight in order that the gypsy's spirit won't try and return.

There are so many rituals which are fascinating to me. For example, the floral tributes are made in the shape of favourite things: the chair she sat in, the pint he drank. Again, they're all designed to keep the 'spirit' happy and away from camp. Everything is done in three's: three days, three weeks, three, six and nine months.

I took a bouquet of peach roses in honour of the many silk ones in her trailer. The morning of the funeral was misty. I parked my car and walked towards an enormous bonfire blazing away in the midst of the clearing. Milling around were hundreds of men. As I approached the crowd divided; it was like the parting of the Red Sea and the whole place went quiet. I was female, non-gypsy, and an official. Just then Elvira spotted me and came running out of her trailer, where the rest of the women had congregated.

'I know her,' she said. 'Come inside, Sally.'

I went inside to pay my respects. Elvira's mother (she was known simply as 'mother') was laid out according to tradition in all her finery, with pennies on her eyes. Apart from the trestle she was laid on, the small caravan had been stripped bare. Her outfit was a traditional gypsy dress of gold embroidery and lace. All the women wear heavy gold jewellery as a way of displaying their wealth and that of their husbands. Together, we stood in silence.

In the autumn of 1996, I began an MSc in Sociology of Health and Welfare at the University of Greenwich. Evening classes were held twice a week and the modules covered child protection, leadership and public health. The two years were a slog but I got my postgraduate diploma. My thesis was based on the death and dying rituals of the gypsies – in many ways it was a tribute to Elvira's family. Shortly after I left the job in 1996 I learned they had moved into houses.

I was a truly contented Mum. Clara, now aged one, was perfectly happy to sit beside me drawing with her crayons and papers. She was an easy child, who slept and ate just as babies should. Highly determined, she reached all her milestones well ahead of schedule. From the age of two, she had clear ideas on what to wear, what to do and how to do it. She chattered away, giving a running commentary on life, her favourite colour (pink), best food (mashed potato) and why dogs were cleverer than cats.

One mystery, however, needed to be cleared up.

Peter and Clara had separate bedrooms. Then we had visitors and so we moved Clara's cot into Peter's room, after which the children refused to go back to separate rooms. Not long afterwards, we often found Clara in the lower bunk of Peter's bed each morning and not in the cot where we had left her at night. Puzzled, we spied on them one evening: Peter got up, dragged the little plastic step over to the cot, helped his sister out of it and tucked her into the lower bunk.

Looking back, I'd say they were wonderful times despite my exhaustion. I'd drive home after work, pick up the kids and spray them with the garden hose to play and cool down in the intense summer heat. Sometimes I was so tired that I would stumble through the front door carrying Clara, three bags, three lunchboxes and my briefcase, unsure of what to tackle first.

In retrospect, I believe the need to do, to take on as much as is humanly possible, is all part of my battle against MS. While I've always been a doer – someone with a plan, a need to set myself a challenge and succeed – the urgency that comes from knowing I'm living with a degenerative disease is a driving force. To everyone who will listen, I say use it because you could lose it: climb that mountain *today*! You don't know what's around the corner: you could wake up tomorrow without the use of your limbs, it's that simple. And while there are lots of MS sufferers who are keen to be informed of every new scientific breakthrough in the hope of finding a cure, I'd much rather get on with the day-to-day: my life, my kids.

In retrospect, I'll admit that the MS was getting worse but I refused to give in to it. Living in the colder climes of Scotland, today I am also aware that heat exacerbates the symptoms. At the same time scientists have found those living nearer the Equator are far less likely to suffer and it's more prevalent in northern Europe where lack of sunlight causes Vitamin D deficiency. Interestingly, at the time of writing the Scottish Parliament is debating whether to give Vitamin D supplements to schoolchildren.

By now, Peter had started at the local primary school. It was a lovely place but they refused to take responsibility for his anaphylaxis (hypersensitivity) or to ban peanuts altogether. Instead I'd have to visit at lunchtimes to check on what he was eating. Eventually, the logistics proved impossible: I simply couldn't get there. And so in January he ended up at a prep school, where they could properly monitor his food and his allergies.

6

Going Home

In March 1997, two years after we moved into Beckenham, Andrew and I went out for supper at our favourite Italian, leaving his mother to babysit. Andrew had been offered a fund management role in Edinburgh. Over the house special (seafood pasta) and a bottle of red, we discussed the pros and cons of the job and taking the family back to Edinburgh. To be honest, there weren't any cons: it had always been part of our 10-year plan, conceived after Peter's birth, to raise our kids in Scotland. We wanted to give them the green hills and the same proximity to the Scottish wilderness and good schools that we'd enjoyed and benefited from as children.

Scotland, in case you've never visited, has an incredible range of landscapes. The white beaches of the North are like a lost Caribbean. Typically they are deserted and you feel cheated if you arrive to find another family already there. 'But this is *our* beach,' you mutter beneath your breath as you set up camp at the opposite end of the bay.

Skye is green and lush while the Cuillins are sharp as witches' teeth – you can't help but think that the English countryside is so bland in comparison with the extremities of Scotland. Most of all, I love the scent of the Highlands: they smell of peat. My favourite whisky is peat-smoked, but now I'm getting carried away.

By the time the dessert trolley arrived (as always, I went for the Tiramisu), we'd raised a glass to the move.

'To Scotland!'

By now, I'd moved to Health Visiting in Orpington, another special venture designed to bring health projects to those in need. It was just a 20-minute drive from home and involved routine part-time health visits. However, the more interesting part of the job was caring for those struck by poverty, unemployment and poor facilities.

As part of my role, I ran an exercise group for depressed mothers. I also organised a breakfast bus for children who would otherwise go to school on an empty stomach and established a support group (with input from Social Services) for parents struggling to cope with their kids for a variety of reasons. My job was enjoyable and our garden now a botanical garden-cum-crèche, crowded with pots and hanging baskets, trees, a rabbit hutch, tricycles and prams. Peter had made friends at school and my MS was relatively under control.

I say *relatively*. In reality, my balance was poor, one leg was numb and I felt permanently exhausted yet I carried on as if nothing was wrong. There were times when I just had to go to bed and sleep, but I couldn't and then there were a few falls but I chose to ignore the pain. Instead I went on as if nothing was wrong.

Finding Harmony

In April 1997, Andrew began his new job and moved up to Edinburgh, where he stayed with his parents in Murrayfield. I remained in Beckenham to allow Peter to finish school. Meanwhile, I felt more and more excited about the prospect of going back to Edinburgh. I hadn't realised how much I'd missed it until I imagined living among those crooked streets in full view of the spires and chimneys of the Old Town. Edinburgh is a higgledy-piggledy city, full of nooks and crannies that open out onto the broad thoroughfare of Princes Street. It has elegant grey stone terraces and the National Monument on Calton Hill: our very own unfinished Parthenon. Framing the view south like an invitation to windswept freedom are the Pentland Hills. They also house a dry ski slope. You can go skiing in the morning and sailing on the Forth in the afternoon.

Our favourite family walk was a slow stroll up to the top of Arthur's Seat. This is the main peak of the group of hills forming Holyrood Park in the centre of the city. It's a wild piece of high land forged from an extinct volcano (approximately 350 million years old), a mile east of the castle. The hill rises 251 metres above the city and it's easy to climb. We used to sit on the top, munching bananas and raisins, while taking in the view. Peter would then run all the way down as Clara happily chatted away. The name, so they say, is based on a legend of King Arthur, which in itself offered plenty of opportunities for storytelling.

So began our new life. Andrew was working Monday to Friday up in Edinburgh and flying down at the weekends, armed with brochures from estate agents. We'd only just finished doing up the house in Beckenham when he suddenly came on the phone to announce excitedly, 'I've found a five-bedroom house. It's detached with a garden; it needs work. I know you haven't seen it, but I want to put an offer in ...' Which was exactly what he did.

I wasn't to see the house until just before our move, during Peter's half term. That May, we drove the kids up to Edinburgh. By this time the children were great long-distance travellers. In the days before electronic gadgetry we relied a lot on storytelling, playing endless rounds of I Spy and making up words from number plates, spotting different coloured cars and of course, that old favourite: counting the number of Eddie Stobart lorries we passed on the road.

Andrew drove us north of the city, past his old school and the Galleries of Modern Art to an area called Black-hall. He turned right into a wide road that I immediately liked: it was leafy and peaceful, with a view of the castle.

'It's the perfect place for watching Hogmanay fire-works,' I told him (and as it turned out, we always end up having a street party. Someone puts the radio on and everyone takes drinks outside).

We pulled up outside a solid detached house with a flowering cherry and two enormous rhododendron bushes in the front. It was white with a Mediterranean feel – the last thing you'd expect of Edinburgh.

'It's very small,' was Peter's first comment.

From a child's perspective it was small because there was no top floor: it's a bungalow. We call it 'the Tardis'.

In fact, it's deceptively big inside and just over 100 years old, with wonderfully high ceilings that give an airy, spacious feel. I'm always amused by the name of the street: Forthview. You can't see the Forth from here but it's a nice idea. However, as we were about to discover, the house was also a real hovel. The previous owners had kept Alsatians and ferrets; they were heavy smokers and everything was stained or painted brown. At least the rooms were large and there was a garden (perfect for a trampoline, sandpit and playing football), with cherry, crab apple, pear and apple trees.

'Can you see the potential?' asked Andrew, glancing at me.

The prospect of doing up another house was daunting. It was as though we were back at the bottom of Everest, preparing for our ascent. *Here we go again*, I thought, preparing myself to live in a building site while a new boiler, gas, electrics, plastering, a paint job, kitchen refurbishment and bathroom installation all took place although of course, we couldn't afford to do everything at once.

'Yes,' I squeezed his hand. 'I can see the potential.'

He smiled.

Just then a neighbour appeared over part of the shared privet hedge to introduce himself.

'Hi, I'm Mark,' he said, 'and I'm absolutely ecstatic you're moving in!'

The previous owners, it seemed, had done nothing to facilitate good neighbourly relations. As soon as we moved in – June 1998 – we immediately had everyone round for tea to introduce ourselves and say hello. They were very welcoming.

Leaving Kent was easy. More of a wrench than anticipated, though, was saying goodbye to friends and my job (I had been in line for promotion and really enjoyed my years there). Our friends from church gave us a photo of the entire congregation and one Sunday afternoon we had a party in the church hall – I had been leader of the youth group, Pathfinders. They gave me a wonderful video with everyone in it: there were images of the church, the congregation and their memories.

There was an interesting smell of rotten egg sandwiches to greet us on arrival in Scotland as Peter's lunchbox was mistakenly packed among the boxes. He was very sad to leave his tree-boat behind! We travelled up separately, arrived before the removal team and then waited and waited. By 7pm, the van still hadn't turned up and eventually they got a message through to let us know that they had broken down. Luckily we were able to spend the night at Andrew's parents' house.

The next day we went to see our new house again and it stank. Layer upon layer of grease had to be scraped off the kitchen and as for the nicotine … well, there was no way we would be moving our children into an ashtray! Instead my long-suffering in-laws let us stay on with them. Over the next three days we went through three bottles of bleach, 10 pairs of rubber gloves and a mountain of wire wool. At that point we could do nothing about the décor, not even the room with Teenage Mutant Ninja Turtles' wallpaper half-painted over, but at least we could remove the stinking carpet and treat the floor below with bleach. Evidently, this was the room in which the ferrets and dog had been left when the owners went out. Eventually we were able to move in.

The next task was to create a happy environment for the kids so that they would feel settled. Upstairs in the loft, Andrew built a bed area for Clara. Afterwards, I put up yellow-and-blue gingham curtains and a canopy over the bed, with drapes that hung down and were secured with big blue ribbons. Andrew made bookshelves with cushions on the top so that Clara could see Edinburgh Castle from her window. Peter had bunk beds: Andrew boarded up the sides and cut out portholes to transform them into a boat. He created a bow with cords attached so Peter could pull them from his bed on the top to create a ferry-like entry. Meanwhile, I made sail curtains and swag-bag cushions. Every night, Peter would lower the bow, climb into bed and set sail for the Land of Nod.

To make ends meet, we took in foreign students, usually two at a time. We had all sorts of nationalities and personalities. There was a crazy Russian boy who only took a shower when I pushed him in and turned on the taps; he wore a sailor cap everywhere. During one evening meal, he stunned us with the announcement: 'When I leave school, I going to be a nuclear officer in Navy!' He shared with a lovely Spaniard, who was eternally patient.

We had students who would chat with us, others who cried. One girl from Mexico managed to max out her new credit card on soft toys during the first week. It transpired that at home she lived in a gated community, with a chauffeur to take her to school. She had never carried money until she was sent to Scotland hence the adventure with the card. We also took in a boy from Mexico whose mother was terrified he would miss his plane (apparently he had a history of it). Despite warnings from us about luggage rules, the students frequently packed at the last minute only to discover that they had overbought and had no space: the number of parcels I had to send on was ridiculous. It was mostly good fun, however, and the children developed a good knowledge of geography and foreign cultures. Meal times were always enjoyable as we encouraged everyone to listen to each other and swap stories.

Peter (who by then was six) began school at The Edinburgh Academy, which we had visited during the May break. His favourite choice, it was a small school that he christened his 'sunshine school' as the sun shone on the day when we went to view. Initially, Clara was at home and then when I started work she attended Mr Squirrels Nursery. Later, aged three, she went to the Edinburgh Academy Nursery.

At the same time as settling in and finding schools and nurseries, I was working part-time as an agency nurse, doing homecare. It was varied and I could choose my own shifts and work when I was able to do so. My favourite job during that time was caring for a famous organist, who was terminally ill. On one of his better days he gave my two-year-old her first piano lesson. He was full of stories and ultimately I gained as much from caring for him as he received. Although I missed my friends and my old job, we were so happy to be in Edinburgh: the children were settled, Andrew was enjoying his new position and we loved being able to jump in the car and escape to the countryside in a matter of minutes.

But then the MS hit with a vengeance. The year we moved up, I had four relapses. When you relapse, you lose something and relapses can last anything from a few days to a few months. This time, I lost the feeling and use of parts of my right side. In the early days they put you on high doses of intravenous steroids over a three-day period. The steroids reduce inflammation, thereby reducing nerve damage. I hated it: as soon as I was hooked up and the steroids began pumping into my body, my mouth filled with a bitter taste that I likened to neat gin. Yes, *disgusting*! After the first session I knew to take in lots of chewing gum and mints, like all the other patients. The treatment leaves you feeling unwell for days, a bit like having chemo without the sickness involved. Latterly, I was given oral steroids, which meant I didn't need to be admitted to hospital. Gradually, over a period of weeks or months, you remit or improve but you never get back what you've lost completely. As a rule you can never recover your physical self – your better self, your *whole* self. Once it's gone, it's gone forever.

While working with the Huntington's Disease Society, I noticed a severe prickling in my right arm; it became so bad that I couldn't use it – I had no control over it. One morning I woke to a nightmare from the past: my right arm wasn't working and I couldn't hold or lift anything.

Clara, now four, was bewildered as I tried to explain why I couldn't brush her glorious waist-length hair. It broke my heart.

'You'll have to brush it this morning, darling,' I told her as gently as I could, talking her through the process. 'That's right. From the top, pull the brush. Yes, you've got it. Now again ...'

A friend drove the kids to school and then it was a case of off to the Western General for more steroids. If you really want to know what it's like, I suggest you tie your hand behind your back to see what you can and can't do. Being unable to do things for myself or others was intensely frustrating: I had to learn to use my left hand ... and fast!

Gradually the sensation in my arm came back but it was very weak, with severe nerve pain. Temporarily, I also lost the ability to speak: my mouth was saggy and my tongue lost its muscle power. Now, as anyone who knows me will tell you, I can talk for Scotland! I talk a lot, too much perhaps. So, not to be able to talk was intensely distressing: bedtime stories, conversations with the children, reassurance, answering the telephone were all impossible. This ushered in more heartache and distress but the steroids and time healed all although one side of my mouth remains a strange shape. My smile is a little lopsided (I think I am the only one who notices, though).

Each time something goes, another bit of the fighting spirit is bashed; your whole being feels battered and bruised. The trouble with MS is that every single part of the body has nerves and so any area can be affected. Like I said, it's a war.

How can I describe it? Imagine putting on a pair of gloves with cut glass inside – that's about it. It was the same sensation with my right foot, as though I was stepping onto cut glass. The pain has never left and is difficult to control – despite the best care, drugs and intentions it is barely under control. All this left me feeling angry and useless but I carried on.

I was overjoyed when, as planned, I became pregnant with our third child. On 6 May 1999, two years after moving back up to Scotland (when the country voted to have its own parliament), I successfully gave birth to our second daughter, Melissa. I enjoyed all my pregnancies. Though tired, I took great pleasure in the knowledge and physical certainty that my body was functioning properly. I'd recovered as much as I could from the relapses and despite my failing health, I was creating new life. Miraculously, the body protects the foetus despite the MS. There had been no indication there would be anything different about this baby. Nor, apart from the emotional lows, was this pregnancy any different to the others besides a serious dose of flu. When I was four months pregnant, I had serious high-temperature and rigours that come with real flu. It started on Boxing Day and by early January I was on a course of antibiotics for a chest infection.

The birth was fast and fabulous. In Edinburgh, I wasn't allowed to deliver in the water but my labour could take place in it. We almost broke the rules and had very little time to get out! As the midwives ripped open sterile packs, there was water everywhere and then out she came. All three of us fell asleep, wrapped up and warm.

Melissa was smaller than my other babies: she weighed 7lb 8oz and I had a bit of a problem with feeding her. Peter and Clara, I'd breastfed ad nauseam – I loved the physical bond and my babies enjoyed my milk. But Melissa was slow to put on weight (just an ounce at a time) and for a mother whose son had fed so much that he put on eight ounces in one week, it came as a shock. I was used to big, thriving babies and so eventually, I ended up supplementing with baby milk to build her up, but still she struggled to suck and feed. I took her home and she joined our high-volume, busy, loving family. Peter and Clara adored their new sister: they were both keen to help and when she finally started on bottles they loved to feed her. We used to joke that Melissa was already capable of making her own decisions ... and taking off. I once came into the kitchen, having left Melissa there, to find an empty room.

'Melissa, Melissa ...'

I began to panic but it turned out that she had rolled underneath the sideboard and was lying there, gurgling away happily.

Then everything changed. The autumn after Melissa was born, I'd gone back to work at the Huntington Disease Society as usual. On a foggy morning on the way to the nursery I took Melissa to the GP for her second set of injections: Diptheria, Tetanus, Whooping Cough and Polio. It's a lot of vaccines to give a small baby, but that's how we do it. It was at an earlier stage than my other two, but the guidelines had changed.

Mid-morning, I received a telephone call from the nursery.

'Sally! Hello, sorry to call,' said the woman in charge of the baby room. 'But something's wrong with Melissa. She's got cold hands and feet and a strange rash.'

Having endured the earlier horror of Peter's anaphylactic shock, I rushed over to the nursery as fast as I could. Melissa was lying in her cot with a bulging fontanelle (the soft spot on her skull) and was covered in red spots. Immediately I drove her back to the GP, where they gave her a shot of antibiotics in case it was meningitis and sent us to the Sick Children's Hospital in an ambulance, blue light flashing. But it wasn't meningitis. In fact, the doctors were unable to make a satisfactory diagnosis and we went home. Melissa recovered from the rash and her body temperature stabilised but as Andrew commented, it was as if someone had flipped a switch: we had another four admissions for the same symptoms of unexplained vomiting, rash and high temperatures. I was overcome with worry and concern, but no one could give me an explanation. What's more, I began to fear the doctors might think that I was doing something to cause my child's strange symptoms. It was all so mysterious.

That summer, we went on holiday to France. Rather than our usual camping, we rented a lovely gîte right at the bottom of Brittany. It was less a holiday than an exercise in endurance as Andrew entertained Peter and Clara while I tried my hardest to comfort Melissa, who screamed and screamed. The fact that she had been such a contented baby made it all the more heart-breaking.

Then she fell silent. For the next six months Melissa said nothing. She did nothing either – my dad called her a 'Russian doll'. Yet no one believed me when I insisted there was a problem. I spent hours putting a rattle in her hand and would shake it to teach her that if she picked it up and shook it, then it would rattle for her. Other times, I would look her in the eye, we would all sing and chat to her or try the physical stimulation of hugs and spinning but all the while there was nothing, no response. Glassy-eyed, she was completely cut-off.

I felt increasingly depressed and coupled with the despair was an anxiety over Melissa's future. In some way I must be to blame for her condition or had, at the very least, exacerbated it, I felt. Later on, when I was able to discuss the events leading up to her change with medical professionals, I realised my responses were similar to a sort of bereavement: shock, disbelief, a sense of being cut off from the world, of no one understanding what it's like to have your child's future taken away. As a fellow parent once said of her own child, it was as if we had packed for one journey and found ourselves at the wrong destination.

Meanwhile, the trauma of Melissa's condition reverberated through our family and put pressure on my relationship with everyone else. Being too young to understand, the elder children were oblivious to my worries and concerns but I was overly tired and continually fought to get help for my youngest. The demands made by a new baby on her mother are always enormous and when the infant has developmental problems too, it's a hundred times worse.

When Melissa was nine months old, I took her to the GP for her nine-month check. I understood the drill and knew what she ought to be doing. After all, I was a mum of three and a health visitor.

'Look,' I said to the health visitor. 'She's not rolling, she's not sitting up, she's not babbling …'

The health visitor, a woman younger than me, did the raisin test. This will be familiar to mums everywhere: does your child have the dexterity to pick up a single raisin? Melissa banged the health visitor's hand.

'I'm not surprised,' observed the health visitor. 'It's a very boring job to ask a little girl to do.'

I wanted to scream. Not only did Melissa not have a pincer grip (the ability to hold something small between her thumb and forefinger), she didn't even have a palmer grip (the dexterity to hold things without using her fingers); she couldn't grip *anything*. She couldn't use her hands. Why wasn't the health visitor taking this lack of motor skills at nine months seriously? Then I went in to see my GP, the same one who had seen me through my pregnancy and treated my other two for the usual coughs and childhood ailments.

'Melissa is at the other end of the scale from your other two,' she told me. 'It's nothing to worry about.' Then turning to Melissa, she said: 'Isn't it a shame? Mummy's got two very bright children and she just wants you to be the same.'

I was appalled. As a health professional, my code of practice has always been to give open and straightforward advice but to listen, too. If you don't pay attention to people's concerns, you will miss the bigger picture. While it's often easier said than done, I can't emphasise enough how isolated this wall of smiles made me feel: it was no good being met with talk of the need for a balanced view. It was – and is – difficult to explain how empty Melissa was. She was completely silent and floppy. However, she seemed to love being sung to and I remember her reacting to a flute concerto playing on the stereo; her eyes sparkled and she waved her hands. Otherwise she just slept and ate what I fed her without demonstrating any physical or emotional change. There were no reactions, no milestones: it was utterly soul-destroying.

In defining abnormal behaviour, it is crucial to understand what's meant by 'normal' behaviour, I already knew that. To me, Melissa's obliviousness to the world around her, her inability to respond or connect, called for a proper assessment. I came away thinking, *I've got to sort this out*. I'd thought that because Melissa was prone to rashes perhaps she had allergies, like Peter, and so I asked my GP for an appointment with a consultant at the Royal Hospital for Sick Children, commonly known as Sick Kids. Eventually, this came through when Melissa was 10 months old. The consultant – a specialist in allergies – didn't believe my story, though.

'Look,' I told him. 'I could leave her on the floor, go out for lunch, come back and she'll be in the same place.'

'Don't knock it,' he said. 'A quiet life must be good. Besides it's quite normal,' he added. 'There's a normal spectrum of behaviour. Development scale is variable.'

Undeterred, I requested a second opinion. This time I would take Andrew as back up. The morning of the second appointment arrived. At my insistence, the consultant agreed to refer Melissa to a physiotherapist. A letter from the consultant (which I was subsequently told about) asked the physiotherapist to please reassure this anxious mother and give her a few ideas and exercises to assist her. The appointment duly arrived and so off we went.

'Look at this,' I said to the physiotherapist, gesturing to Melissa, whose fists were clenched up around the sides of her head.

'It's all right,' she told me. 'I've seen …'

I put Melissa face down on the floor. There she would have remained until she suffocated, had I not picked her up. This was not the normal response of a one-year-old. The physiotherapist immediately referred us to a neurologist, which was when they started to believe us. And so began twice-weekly physiotherapy sessions, followed by years of weekly home visits as Melissa learned to sit and unclench her fists. At the age of one, she had the gross motor skills of a three-month-old baby. As the initial diagnosis of Global Neurodevelopmental Delay (she was in fact developmentally delayed and they didn't have a name for it) was made, it dawned on me just how far we – and above all, Melissa – had to go.

7

Black Days

'They're better off without me.'

Through the window I could see the seagulls circling the tops of trees. The counselling room of the Post Natal Depression Project was on the fourth floor of a Victorian redbrick in the centre of Edinburgh. Every week, I'd force myself back into that wicker chair by the window, the one with the pretty cushions. I'd look out at the garden, away from my hands twisting the same soggy bit of tissue. If I wanted to scream, I would gain control by looking at the sky; when it got too painful, I could soar into the clouds.

I was desperate: desperate for sleep, desperate for help, desperate for respite from the day-to-day struggle of looking after three small children. Caring for Melissa, supporting her needs, had brought me to my knees; I felt drained. Every day was a battle to find the will to go on. I just wanted to understand what was going on inside Melissa's head – and mine. Sylvia Plath's image of being stuck under a bell jar is right: I couldn't find a way out. Salvador Dalí has a painting of a woman's splintered head (the missing bits are balls circling her head) so apt it took my breath away when I first saw it.

While pregnant with Melissa, I'd voiced my worst fears to my GP and my health visitor. I admitted that I was terrified of developing post-natal depression.

'We'll keep an eye on you,' they insisted.

In one of the antenatal classes for groups of mums with kids that I attended, where you talk about past experiences and fears, one woman mentioned her experience of post-natal depression and the amazing support offered by the Post Natal Depression Project. I'd also touched on my brief experience of depression. After the class, the other mum gave me their number.

One warm afternoon when I was pregnant with Melissa and feeling very down, I called the number. I chatted briefly to a woman who offered to arrange for me to come and see them.

But I never went, and then I had Melissa. Looking back, I realise that I must have been depressed immediately after her birth: I felt overwhelmed by life and by my MS. I remember my Aunty Pat and Uncle Andy visiting me and taking Melissa out so that I could rest but instead I paced the floor, scarcely able to breathe: I was desperately anxious to have her back yet I also wanted someone to take her away, to give me a break. Strange. Only when I look back do I see my anxiety was muddled with certainty there was something wrong with Melissa.

In January 2000 my world collapsed. Six months after Melissa was born, I'd gone back to work as a nurse for the Huntington's Disease Society. Huntington's Disease is a progressive neurodegenerative disorder that leads to dementia and is far more common than widely perceived. Many families hide the truth of their loved ones' suffering, which means deaths from the disease go incorrectly recorded. My job was to provide those families with support, advice and practical help; I was there for anyone affected by the disease.

However, at work I felt very unsupported. What's more, it seemed to me that I wasn't juggling home and work commitments at all well. Then I got a bad chest infection and so I was off sick. Around this time, Melissa had another of her strange illnesses (an unexplained rash and fever), which meant she had to go into hospital. Frantic with worry, I called work to let them know that I wouldn't be able to come in and my team leader was so rude that I put the phone down and rang my GP instead.

'I can't cope,' I told her. 'I can't do this anymore!'

'Come and see me,' she said gently.

I refused anti-depressants but she gave me time off work.

'I can't face going back to work,' I told Andrew.

My husband had recently completed an MBA and knowing me so well, said he would fund me for a year to set up my own business and so I started up an au pair agency. Now you have to remember that before most of Eastern Europe was invited to join the EU, there were slim-pickings when it came to finding au pairs in Edinburgh. You were offered girls from Italy, Spain and France but most of them wanted to stay in London to go nightclubbing and shopping on Oxford Street. Bouncing

Melissa with one hand, stirring bolognaise with the other, I was on the phone all day talking to prospective au pairs and clients. In a frenzy of activity, I set up the computer in the kitchen (I didn't even know how to switch it on at first) and had to learn how to download files, create documents and send emails. Rather than ignore the phone, I took every call too.

'*Bonjour.*'

'*Buenos dias.*'

'*Buongiorno.*'

In between answering the telephone, interviewing French, Spanish and Italian girls using my basic language skills – not to mention all the Eastern bloc girls who were desperate to get UK visas – I was struggling with my MS symptoms of wobbly legs plus a dodgy arm and eye. In retrospect, it's easy to say I took on too much but I've never been the type to turn down an opportunity and at the time it seemed like a good opportunity. In keeping busy, I hoped the sense of emptiness, the loneliness, would just go away.

But I couldn't relax into being a mum: I felt guilty about all the things I couldn't do, and wasn't doing. Always, I felt as if I should be doing more. I wasn't sure what exactly that might be, but I learned to live with two heads: the anxious, terrified one and the 'we're managing well' one. It was as if I was running through a dark forest, then stumbled and was about to trip, the branches tearing at my hair. I had to keep moving, I had to protect the children – I couldn't see any light or patches of grass. Andrew, meanwhile, was totally supportive but didn't really see how busy I was, as it all happened when he was at work.

Later on, I admitted that the smarter, more together I looked, the worse I actually felt. I'd put on my make-up and best clothes and go off to appointments, struggling in a pit of despair. The only exception to the rule was counselling, which I often attended in a baggy tracksuit with unkempt hair. Andrew, meanwhile, was working hard and I didn't want to burden him with it. Of course in the end he noticed my moods but there was nothing much he could do.

To outward appearances, I was a fully functioning wife and mother as well as a businesswoman. I never missed a parents' meeting or a musical performance and I always told the children how much I loved them. We baked, we read stories: in fact, I used to *make up* stories. Peter's were about dinosaurs in a magical world where good little boys slid down dinosaur tails into a moat of jelly and ice cream, with balloons flying overhead. Clara's were filled with longhaired mermaids swimming through underwater caves alongside princesses wearing beautiful jewels.

I hid my darkness. On bad days, I'd wake up and think, *OK, I've got 12 hours until I can get back into bed.* Andrew was hugely patient with me but he was also working long hours and depression, by its very nature, is introspective: it draws you in until you've lost sight of the outside world.

After the birth of Clara, the GP in Beckenham had offered anti-depressants but I refused them and over time, my OCD faded. This time it was worse for everything was intensified: we would get out of the car, start walking up the road to school and I'd ask the kids to go back to check the handbrake was on and the doors were locked. I couldn't leave the house without going back inside to make sure the oven and the light switches were turned off. I'd have to change Melissa's outfit because of a mark on the front; then I'd change my shirt because I too had a mark on my front – by which time, I'd be in a panic about time. And then the phone would ring.

To this day, I can't hear the sound of a phone ringing without experiencing a Pavlovian response. A bolt of fear rips through me: *has one of the au pairs done something wrong? Will the host family sue me? Could I be sent to prison? Will the kids be taken from me?* I paid huge amounts of liability insurance. In the end, after a very successful three years two things destroyed the business: my health deteriorated and the EU opened up. Today, the girls find their own jobs. Eventually, I said goodbye to the business and passed it on in 2007.

When I finally knocked on the door of the Post Natal Depression Project run by Crossreach Post Natal Depression Services in early 2000, I had reached the very bottom. I can't say why I knocked on the door on that particular day but all I knew was if I didn't get help – and soon – I'd be consumed by my fears. I didn't want them to affect the children anymore than they already had.

The waiting room was full of comfy chairs and well-thumbed copies of *Hello!* and *Good Housekeeping*, with women trying not to look at each other. No one ever spoke – I guess we were all too wrapped up in our own pain, embarrassment and shame.

What had happened to make us feel as if we were unfit mothers?

I had my first meeting with an extremely experienced counsellor, a lovely woman with a gentle smile who always looked reassuringly poised and professional in coordinated outfits that complimented her reddish hair. At the initial consultation to see if the Project could help, I was exceedingly fortunate: I was offered assistance the moment I asked. Today there is a long waiting list for the service. We chatted about my family, where the kids went to school, my life and daily routine. At this stage, I was feeling far too overwhelmed to talk about my MS but it wasn't long before my counsellor worked it into our sessions.

My counsellor had a great sense of humour. It was useful for me to have someone who had a Christian faith although there wasn't an overtly religious message behind her counselling. Immediately, I warmed to her: she didn't have the stereotypical breathy, soft voice I'd imagined a counsellor might have. Strong and tough, she was prepared for a challenge and there was nothing wishy-washy about her. And she wouldn't take no for an answer: she couldn't be manipulated into believing all was well when it obviously wasn't – she was only interested in the truth.

At the same time, I felt that I could really open up and talk to her about everything. I told her about my MS and how I overcompensated for my illness by trying to make everything perfect. I'd wake to find the kitchen was a tip and the living room a nightmare but the whole place would be cleaned perfectly by the time the kids went to school. I told her about the trap door in my head that I had to keep shut to keep the pain away. The trouble was, it kept springing open because the space above was too full. Throughout my sessions, Andrew was supportive in the background but as an extremely private person, he felt uncomfortable with the process.

My OCD was spiralling: by then I had no patience and I'd lost all sense for perspective. When one of Peter's primary school teachers said he was lazy (he was just seven years old), I accepted this without argument. At the parents' night, we were virtually dismissed without anything said. His teacher listed all the negatives and then bid us goodbye before we could answer back. In any case, both Andrew and I were far too shell-shocked and exhausted by this point to say anything. That night, I cried buckets. Was it true? If so, it must be my fault – I had too much going on at home. Indeed, life was spent juggling the business, helping Melissa, getting homework done with the two older kids, hiding my fears about the MS and trying not to overreact to daily situations that would frequently send me into a panic.

I was suffering such emotional pain and I felt that I wasn't spending enough time with Peter. Meanwhile, he was being bullied. Within a week of him starting at senior school it was dealt with and never recurred, but during his junior-school years he suffered. You can never repair that damage: the failure to intervene and stick up for your child.

Recently, I tried to talk to Peter about it.

'Oh Mum, move _on_! That was years ago. I'm fine,' he insisted. 'It's not a problem.'

He is still my little soldier. Our children have since grown up and moved on: every day they amaze me with their achievements and lust for life.

Clara's Primary 1 teacher was a woman called Ali, who has since become a close friend and a great support. One day, Clara and I were walking across the playground when she went full tilt across the asphalt. There I was with my gammy leg, baby Melissa and now Clara was bawling in pain with scraped knees and hands.

'Stop crying,' I said gently, trying to comfort her.

But I couldn't pick her up – I didn't have the physical strength. Instead I felt crushed and panicked by my uselessness. A kind mum took the baby. We walked into school and she handed Melissa over to Ali, who had rushed out to help. She took us to the medical room and left Clara and me alone. Finally, I was able to deal with my daughter's cuts and grazes, to give her all the cuddles she needed while trying not to burst into tears myself. I felt such a failure and the memory of her fall, the thought of how I wanted to respond and couldn't still haunts me; it's a huge sadness.

In contrast, her memory of that moment is one of cuddles and Mummy making it all better. Once again, I am so proud of my kids.

Finding Harmony

The Project ensured the counselling was regular weekly sessions and they didn't charge for their services, they had a collection box instead. On days when I could barely climb out of bed, let alone get dressed and into town to discuss why I couldn't leave my bed, they would send a taxi to the house. I'd arrive and one of the project leaders, would greet me at the door with a great big smile.

'You look well today.'

It was a kind thing to say. Despite my tracksuit, plimsolls and unkempt hair, it made me feel better too. I'd hand over Melissa, who was taken to the crèche, and take a sweet mug of tea.

I didn't let go of that mug; indeed, nothing in the world would have induced me to do so. Clutching it with both hands, I took it upstairs to the counselling room and only after I started to talk and the pain eased did I feel able to put the mug down. Ignoring the clock on the coffee table telling me that my time was running out, I'd take a tissue from the box of Kleenex For Men and blow my nose.

I was determined to get better, despite my misgivings. Andrew must have needed to draw on his reservoir of patience, though: I would tell him I'd been to counselling and sometimes what I had worked through. Typically, however, my conversations with the counsellor remained a confidential matter: I had to do the healing myself. Andrew was always there for me but he couldn't fight my demons. I tried really hard to make sure things were organised and settled when he got home from work, that the kids were happy and we were playing. Life appeared under control.

But it took a long time to recover. Boy, was it painful! I hated exposing my thoughts yet I also relished the support of the counsellor. The Project had a crèche run by fantastic workers who cared for Melissa and could see her behaviour for themselves; they supported me while she was going through the tests and was ultimately diagnosed. Also, I knew that they believed my story and they listened to me, which was a huge help.

I came to dread the end of each session: I'd walk away from the house down the long drive feeling as though I'd been tossed out into the world to fend for myself. Already I'd feel the loss of my counsellor's reassuring voice, the loss of the building itself; I felt safe there with someone to look after Melissa and someone to listen to me. I'd get in the car, turn the key in the ignition and feel utterly, hopelessly alone. And I couldn't leave without glancing back at the building, knowing they had moved on to help the next depressed mum.

I'd been forgotten. I hated everyone, I resented being abandoned – how dare they?

One day I woke to find the sun had gone out: everything was black. I had reached the depths of my despair and could no longer see a way through the depression clouding me for so long; I just wanted it all to end.

The big kids went off to school and with Melissa beside me, I sat down at the kitchen table and wrote an account of my despair. Afterwards I fed Melissa and put her in the car. I had a counselling session at 11am, after which I'd been asked to take my grandmother from Fife to hospital.

Somehow the knowledge that I knew what to do brought a sense of incredible calm; I felt calmer than in months. Now the raging storm had subsided: I was to end the pain for everyone and the world would be a better place without me.

'How are you today?' asked the counsellor, waiting for me to arrange myself on the chair.

I crossed my legs, uncrossed them and fixed my gaze on the tree straight ahead. It had shed all its leaves.

'I've got a plan,' I told her. 'I'm going to take Paracetamol, go to the Forth Road Bridge and jump off it.'

This was all quite matter of fact: indeed, I felt a sense of icy calm. She listened and nodded, then began talking – lots and lots of things that I don't remember. Then through the fog of words came the mention of my son's name: *And what would that teach Peter about coping? How will he cope when things get tough if this is what his mother has taught him?*

I was furious: I hated her for doing this to me – for using guilt and motherhood to stop me leaving them. At the end, I left the session seething. Though I still had 'The Plan', I knew in the back of my mind she had won.

What will the children learn from this?

Her words echoed round and round my head as I got into the car. I collected the other children from school, cooked sausages and mash and somehow carried on with day-to-day living. In retrospect, my counsellor was reminding me of all the things I'd said in past sessions about wishing to be a positive role model for my kids; I wanted to teach them how to deal with things in an optimistic way. She was reiterating *my* words.

The next session was rocky. I was still angry – in fact, I filled another two pages with bitter words about how I felt. What's more, I resented my counsellor's emotional tone and was furious with her for talking me down.

'Why did you let me go?' I demanded to know.

I made her listen to what I'd written, repeating how angry I felt.

'I knew it was safe,' she told me. 'The alternative would have been to keep you here, to have you sectioned and call Andrew.'

With all her experience she had felt certain that I wouldn't do something stupid and she was right. Ironically, this was the start of my recovery. She persuaded me that I really did need anti-depressants and so we struck a deal. She would commit to being my personal counsellor while I took the medication. Recovery was long and protracted but gradually we increased the distance between appointments from weekly to fortnightly and I slowly reduced the anti-depressants. Finally, after too many years I left counselling in 2003.

'You're the only one left that needs to forgive Sally,' were some of the last wise words she said to me.

I never went back for the last session, I just couldn't – I didn't want to force the final severance. Every week I'd find an excuse not to go until six months became a year and it was evident enough time had passed for both sides to acknowledge we had reached the end of our path. However, I'm proud to say that one year on, I chaired a committee and we held a fundraising ball for the Bluebell Project (as the PND project had been renamed). It was a great success and made me see how far I'd come and how well I was. Now it was time to move on from those dark days but I will always remember the people who helped me through.

8

Fighting for Melissa

I was now committed to getting Melissa to the next stage: I wanted all the normal things for her, or at least some of them. At the recommendation of Caroline, a friend whose daughter is severely physically disabled, I took her to Bridgwater's Brainwave – a fantastic charity in Somerset that is dedicated to helping anyone with any sort of brain injury who can benefit from cognitive and physical exercise programmes. 'Brain injury' doesn't have to be the result of an accident but can be due to illness, birth or genetics; the definition is intentionally wide. The charity has purpose-built units for those who have to travel long-distance and need somewhere to stay.

Andrew was on business in London and so I drove down with Melissa (our other two were looked after by their grandparents and the au pair) and he came across by train; we picked him up from the station. It was a very hot day. That evening, with Melissa in her 'Major Buggy' – a sort of pushchair for bigger children with mobility issues – we took a lovely stroll beside a canal. Afterwards we enjoyed a pub meal during which Melissa was royally entertained by ducks and hens in the garden. Again, we had found an oasis of green. We also did a walk in the Chiltern Hills that day, which raised our spirits.

The next day – Assessment Day – came and with it an endless round of questions followed by discussion. Afterwards they videoed Melissa attempting various tasks and more questions; we had a break for lunch and yet more analysis of Melissa and her abilities. We were asked what we would like to gain for Melissa. I found the process increasingly difficult because of her visible distress; they needed Melissa to try the tasks to see what she could (and couldn't) do, but the pressure of having to do them upset her. It transpired because she hadn't started crawling, part of her brain was not properly developed; she also had weak cheek and mouth muscles. Her responses to pain were delayed and she was intolerant of noise and textures. Both of us found the questions and analysis difficult but also reassuring as this was something we could do for Melissa and already, the observations were proving helpful to us.

The following day we were shown a series of exercises devised by the physiotherapists and child development workers and taken through them. After lunch, we had to do the programme while being videoed and then we were shown the video and given the equipment we needed, including a wobble board (a square plastic board with a cylinder underneath that enables it to rock, or wobble). Following this, we were sent on our way with a copy of the exercise programme and video for the volunteers.

Six days out of seven, Melissa spent an hour on the programme with an amazing bunch of volunteers. Together we practised all sorts of exercises to stimulate sensation in her face and uncurl her hands. We had paintbrushes and washing pads (the green-backed kind) that we used to stroke upwards on both sides of her face and round her mouth. Her hands were permanently curled due to developmental delay. One by one, we uncurled her fingers and again used brushes to rub backwards and forwards across her palms. A lot of time was spent on the floor. We rolled Melissa like a pencil, backwards and forwards, across a mat to trigger the workings of her brain. She was encouraged to mimic the volunteers crawling and rolling but she hated it and cried, which for a mum was equally distressing.

We then sang songs, which she loved. It transpired she could cope better with the exercises if we sang and so we rolled to 'Row, Row, Row the Boat'. We swung her from side to side to 'Side to Side, Rocking and Swaying' and did the wobble-board to 'This Is the Way the Lady Rides'. What a fantastic group they were! The majority turned out to be friends of my parents-in-law who had responded to a poster campaign asking for volunteers (they still see Melissa when she visits their church with her granny and granddad).

Andrew and I then did the same programme most evenings; we also got started on the physiotherapy exercises. It was hard work but we were rewarded by seeing Melissa slowly improve in confidence and being cheeky and non co-operative – at last she could voice her own opinions.

Finding Harmony

Already we had had one break-through with Melissa, which had given us hope when we went camping on the Costa Brava the summer before attending Brainwave. We flew to Barcelona, picked up a rental car and gazed out at turquoise waters as we drove in search of a hidden spot. It felt wonderful to be in Spain and we found just what we were looking for in Rosas. We had pre-booked a static tent with raised beds so that I could get in and out easily, as could Melissa. It was a small campsite. Our tent was underneath a tree, which was the only bit of green for miles around. Everything was hot and sandy.

For me the best thing about camping is the sense of freedom and cooking outdoors. You could smell the wild rosemary. Every evening as the sun went down, Andrew would open a bottle of wine and we would watch the older kids chase lizards while Melissa looked on happily. Some evenings, they went to the entertainment run by the campsite. Our tent was only five minutes away from a whirlwind of discos, talent shows and fancy-dress competitions. Peter and Clara both won first prize with the costumes I made them from bits and pieces found in the tent: Peter was James Bond, while Clara was a hula-hula girl.

It was that kind of balmy evening when our miracle happened. The German couple opposite us had a dog; the man was a paediatrician and they had slightly older kids. Between us was a dusty track. Melissa spotted their dog, a Lassie-type Collie, and pulled herself up on a chair. With the aid of the chair, she took her first step and her gaze didn't leave the dog.

'Look!' I nudged Andrew.

I saw the wife nudge her husband as Melissa took one, two, three … and finally six steps across the track before she collapsed onto the dog. There wasn't a dry eye in the house. I was crying, the woman opposite was crying and Andrew was pretending not to cry! And then Peter and Clara came back and they were so excited.

The next day we took Melissa to the beach, where we quickly discovered the sand was too hot for her feet. We went to the beach shop where they sold sun umbrellas and ice creams, and bought her first pair of sandals: a red pair of Jellys. Up until then she'd worn all sorts of boots with inserts and splints. Melissa never liked shoes but she *loved* those Jellys. We have a wonderful photo of her taking her first steps in sand – which is tricky when you've only just mastered the art of standing upright. She was over two years old by then but so small she looked like a one-year-old.

Before you could say sangria, it was time to yank out the tent pegs, drop the guy ropes, pack up and go home. Shivering beneath grey skies, we disembarked at Edinburgh airport and I realised, *wow, I'm about to turn 40!* In the madness of life, it was a milestone I could easily have missed. *So I'd made it to 40: I had to do something. So, what did I do?*

I climbed Ben Ptarmigan, of course. By now I felt a change in my body: physically, things were harder. No one used the term 'secondary progressive' until a couple of years after I'd turned 40 but as ever, I knew. For me, climbing mountains has always meant exactly that:

getting to the top. In my forty-first year I wanted to reach the top of Ben Ptarmigan and look out at the view, to feel the wind on my face and the air whistling past my ears. The only problem was my legs. Would they get me there? It was doubtful. My most recent relapse, eight months prior to this, had triggered a severe deterioration, ending the ability to walk unaided. I knew this could be my last chance, my last challenge, before the winds of change pushed me towards Zimmer frames and wheelchairs.

'Don't worry,' said Andrew. 'I'll get you up there.'

Preparing for the walk was like getting ready for a battle campaign. My parents-in-law had the three children for the day. Andrew deliberately picked Ben Ptarmigan so that we could park at the bottom and there wasn't a long walk in. My brother-in-law Richard (who is four years younger than Andrew) accompanied us and so with sturdy arms on either side of me, I set off on a windy, sun-dappled day.

Ben Ptarmigan is the sort of Munro where you think you can see the top from the very beginning but as you get closer comes the realisation that it's a false summit: you have to go down before you can go up. My right foot kept catching on the heather. As I progressed, I relied more and more on Andrew and Richard, as well as my trusty 'Leki' (a special walking stick for hill walkers).

After we reached the top, smelt the wild heather and gulped from the water bottle, I called home to say: 'I'm at the top!'

Turning to Andrew, I said: 'Couldn't you have found me an easier one?'

'You wouldn't have wanted an easier one!' he laughed. Later it transpired there was a track on the other side that would have taken me part of the way but Andrew knew I wouldn't go for that. And he was right. I remember feeling utterly exhausted from the climb down: my adrenalin levels had faded and it was just a hard slog. Also, I felt sad – a feeling I kept to myself as I didn't want to seem ungrateful but I knew this would be the last Munro that I would reach the top of. On the way back to Edinburgh, we stopped for pints of real ale to celebrate what a triumph it had been.

My worst fears were confirmed by the consultant neurologist at The Western General Hospital who sent me for an MRI scan in June 2003 – 'You really wouldn't want to be stuck in there with a wasp!' joked Andrew. My consultant told me that I was now suffering secondary progressive MS. This is characterised by a more steady progression of symptoms and fewer relapses, just downhill all the way, and it tends to occur in MS sufferers over the age of 40 (I describe it as my war wounds playing up). As the brain is no longer able to continue to compensate for the faulty bits caused by damage to the nervous system, the damage already done worsens. I remember feeling angry and determined this wouldn't happen to me as if I had any choice in the matter.

Melissa's world (and mine too) had become medicalised to the point where I didn't know who was doing what. If it wasn't so ridiculous, it might have been funny. From 2002 onwards, trying to read my diary was a nightmare – I'd have to double-check everything.

'Physio': Is that me or Melissa? 'Neurologist': Melissa or me?

And then at the age of four, Melissa started at nursery, an educational nursery founded by the education department. The first educational psychologist we had in Edinburgh was a wonderful, no-nonsense lady called Patsy, who came to see us to discuss early years provision. She sent me to The Cottage in Edinburgh. The centre was set up to provide therapy for children from birth to the age of three and is run by Capability Scotland, the leading disability charity. We continued to go there twice a week for the next two years but what I really needed to find was a nursery. Patsy suggested Abbey Hill, a nursery with speech and language therapy, and it was perfect. All the children learn how to sign. As important as the emphasis on speech therapy is the physical layout of the nursery. Melissa was, and still is prone to claustrophobia but Abbey Hill has high ceilings and lots of outdoor space. At last, she began to thrive.

Peter and Clara reciprocated Melissa's sense of achievement and her pride in being able to communicate for they became her speech therapy assistants. They taught her how to roll her tongue around sounds, to stress consonants and would wait for a response from her or make her indicate which mug she wanted to drink from. They were great. Words are secret doorways to the world and at last, they could communicate with their little sister and share the experience of life. For years she had been mute, doll-like even. Now she could answer back and demand biscuits and juice (a facility of which she made full use). She was part of the gang!

Melissa particularly loved the singing sessions. She would clap and laugh. It was another opportunity for her to relate to Peter and Clara, whose lives had become dominated by music in a way I'd never imagined possible although perhaps dreamed of. To see your children perform Handel's Messiah or the Stabat Mater in a choir is a magical experience; it's incredible. For our family, music had become a way of life.

My children's talents had first been discovered and encouraged by their inspirational music teachers and new paths seemed to open daily. By the age of 11, Peter was learning the French horn and singing with the National Children's Choir. He had a very energetic music teacher at school who took the boys under her wing and inspired them to great things: Sheena Graham encouraged his talents from the moment he arrived.

Clara, in the meantime, had picked up Peter's French horn and begun to play. I was standing in the living room with Sheena, who had come to give Peter an extra lesson at home when we were interrupted by a halting rendition of 'Mary Had a Little Lamb'.

'That's very unusual,' said Sheena as we both turned, stunned, to see seven-year-old Clara blowing into the horn. 'You should do something with that.'

And so I did. To give you a bit of history, I had a musical education in the sense of having learnt the piano and cello but I play both in a fumbling sort of way. I have strong memories of lying in bed, listening to Mum playing Beethoven's Symphonies at floor-shaking volume as she studied for her degree in geography at St Andrew's. We lived in Fife, which is close to Edinburgh. My parents always made a huge effort to take me to ballets, operas and orchestral performances. For my twelfth birthday, I was escorted to *La Bohème* and shed buckets when the heroine died of consumption.

But Andrew is the musical one. I should also mention here that Andrew, his brother Richard and both our fathers sing beautifully and have been members of choirs at various stages in their lives. As a boy, Andrew sang in the school choir and in our respective churches. For him, singing is something that he really enjoys and sadly, rarely has time for. It was not unusual for me to go out and return to find some huge choral piece blasting away on the stereo with Andrew, joined by Clara, singing the respective lines.

Andrew has the musical genes that my lucky children have inherited and particularly now, it seems, Clara. Following the French horn incident, we talked to the music teacher at Clara's school, who invited her to visit the music department and try out various instruments.

'Mum, Mum, I love the trumpet!' she ran out to tell me.

Trumpet? Where did that come from? Indeed, Clara proved so able that in a very short space of time she was playing alongside 20 other girls. There was one music stand, apparently abandoned: in fact it was where Clara was sitting (she was so small that you couldn't see her). She was the little mascot behind her stand.

Fighting for Melissa

When Clara turned seven, we went to an open morning at St Mary's music school in Edinburgh New Town. There, we were given a tour by some of the older pupils. At the end of it, Clara burst into tears and said, 'I *have* to go to this school – there's music wherever you go!'

At that point, we were encouraged to think about a chorister place. St Mary's was where Clara's musical talents were encouraged in earnest and where she began to excel. As a chorister there was an intensive singing regime. The choir would sing from Monday to Friday at 8.15am, school began at 9.45am and then there was choir tea at 4.30pm, followed by a service at 5pm. On Sundays, they sang twice. They were very long days for Clara. I remember dropping her off in her formal uniform of grey skirt, white shirt, tie and blazer over which she wore bright red cassocks. Turning to the au pair at the time, I asked: 'Am I doing the right thing?'

'Look how happy she is,' came the reply.

Clara herself never had a moment's doubt: she loved it. For me it was proof that despite my MS and depression and Melissa's problems, both my older children were enjoying a happy home life while excelling at school and in their music. The day when Clara got her surplice (the white overlay that went on top of the cassock to signify she was no longer 'in training') was a special moment. In her five years at St Mary's she sang in live broadcasts on the BBC and in services that were recorded – we have all the CDs she was in too.

One evening when I was saying goodnight, Clara asked: 'Why do they have all these services when sometimes there's only one person in the congregation?' I said: 'You have to think of it as part of a bigger community: if you imagine all the services taking place across the country at the same time, then you get a sense of their significance.' It was then that Clara explained her belief system to me.

'I speak to Jesus at home and God in the cathedral,' she told me.

From then on she would have a list of people to pray for each day. She sometimes challenged the clergy on their sermons too, which I always found amusing.

Clara's new school and role as a chorister was interesting for me spiritually: I'd been used to evangelical churches. Now we decided to worship as a family and so we moved to the cathedral. To be honest, I went in with a slightly cynical attitude. I had no expectations, yet I discovered that the music – Benjamin Britten's 'Missa Brevis for Three Trebles' – had a similar calming effect to nature. Listening to the liturgy and the choir music was truly uplifting, a balm to the soul. To be able to gaze up at the new stained-glass window designed by Eduardo Paolozzi and the enormous cross painted with red poppies after World War I and suspended from the roof and feel the sense of history and closeness to God and my family eclipsed everything that had happened during the week.

Gradually, I would feel my mood lift: the tension in my shoulders disappeared and I'd be transported to a place where everything made sense. I'd also found Dean and Jane, two members of the clergy who made sense of my faith. Dean continues to be my spiritual director, for which I'm very grateful – it's some journey!

In her last year Clara became one of two head choristers and skilled at playing the *clàrsach* (a small Scottish harp, wire-strung and a joy to listen to). Eventually she stayed on at St Mary's as an instrumentalist which she started in the autumn of 2009 and still attends the same school.

Music is at the heart of our family: whatever our differences, it's where we meet. At Christmas 2009, Andrew, Clara and Peter swelled the ranks in the choir of Dean's church (he has since moved on from the cathedral). To hear my three singing and practising together was wonderful – all they needed was an alto and unfortunately my voice didn't quite hit the right spots!

Music was Clara's choice: we didn't want to be pushy parents. The guiding principle in her musical upbringing and education had to be that we followed her lead. Unlike other children, she and her friends *wanted* to practise. In fact, we were told by the school to discourage excessive practice for fear of ruining their muscles. It was incredible to know that I happened to be the mother of a gifted child, yet somehow this gift seemed to fit with my life.

9

Night Falls

We were in the car, driving through Wales: to give Melissa a holiday, we were staying with our friends Huw and Ali while Andrew and Clara were on a tour of the States and Canada with the cathedral choir (Peter was with Granny and Grandad Edinburgh, Andrew's parents).

Things were desperate.

In the summer of 2008 Melissa's still-undiagnosed autism manifested itself in such a way that in retrospect was proportionate to her age. As she grew, so did her autism. Some behavioural tics were new while others were an exaggeration of present symptoms that up to that point I hadn't given much thought to. All day and every day, she panicked at the slightest disturbance. If the phone rang or there was a knock at the door, she jumped; if she heard a siren miles away she would start screaming. She liked things to be exactly the same and change upset her. If I said we were going to the zoo and would then have lunch, we couldn't do it the other way round; we would have to do the activity as planned. She would only wear clothes in certain combinations and if one top was dirty, no way was she going to wear the trousers that, to her mind, went with the top.

By now Melissa had become obsessed with attempting to rub out the lines on her hands and constantly tried to rub them on her face and teeth; she was also preoccupied with water and incessantly washed her hands. If she's anxious, she rubs her nose – it's her first sign of distress. At least now we can spot it and intervene; she rubs it so hard that she can cause her nose to bleed and she's terrified of blood. Well, you can see the vicious cycle: for Melissa, life was a trauma and as parents, it was upsetting to witness this.

Much later when an autism specialist likened the condition to being stuck in a burning building, I immediately grasped the gravity. You can't talk to autism sufferers when they panic because they're experiencing such high levels of fear and adrenalin; they're terrified.

Huw and Ali live near Swansea and they're a great support to Melissa, who adores them both. They are incredibly kind and even adapted their house to accommodate our needs. We were on our way to a day out at a farm park, a big treat, when Huw put on his Seekers' CD. Melissa loves The Seekers – we used to play their CD all the time at home and sing along, rocking, rolling, riding.

'I'm going to be sick, I'm going to be *sick*!' Melissa started to scream.

We had to stop the car. Fortunately there was a public toilet near the lay-by. Melissa bolted into the disabled cubicle and began washing and drying her hands in an attempt to calm herself. After ten minutes of this (I didn't try to stop her), she was sufficiently calm to get in the car again but the CD had to be put away.

Our Seekers' CD at home was a studio recording whereas Huw's version turned out to be a live audience with The Seekers: people were clapping and talking, the songs were acoustic. Spot the difference. This is what we were living with, this is how extreme it was but still we had no diagnosis. In April of that year at Melissa's annual check-up the community doctor for children with special needs was of the view that there were characteristics matching autism. The doctor was also concerned about her need for rigid routines and mounting obsessions. Some were OK, such as her thing about monkeys. I've lost count of the number of soft toy monkeys she had – we once had a hugely successful holiday in Dorset where we went to Monkey World all day, every day.

Our lives were defined by attempts to pacify Melissa and stop her screaming. It was a full-time job. One evening I told her that Dad and I were going to Clara's concert and Peter would be babysitting. I gave her a kiss and drove to the school, where I'd arranged to meet Andrew. By now he was working as a regeneration consultant down in London and had been delayed at work. Rather than arrive at Clara's recital three-quarters of the way through, he'd driven straight home. He unlocked the door.

'Hi, it's me,' he called out.

Melissa rushed into the hall and started screaming. Now when I say screaming, I mean hysterical screaming.

She couldn't articulate why she was screaming nor could she stop. (Obviously, it was because Andrew was supposed to be at the concert but had come home early.) Later on, he admitted to me that he had been tempted to leave the house again but where was the logic in that? One of the ways in which we cope with Melissa's screaming is by *not* talking to her. This is in line with the autism specialist's guidelines: her levels of fear and adrenalin are so advanced at this stage that to try and have a conversation is futile.

In the morning, Andrew got up and left for work at his usual time of 6.30am. He'd gone by the time Melissa appeared, bleary-eyed, in our bedroom and got into bed with me for a cuddle.

'Look,' she said, pointing to the empty side of the bed. 'Dad *did* go to the concert!'

For Melissa, mornings start badly if she's had a particularly vivid dream. She has a limited perception of how her mind works and identifying subtle differences in thoughts and feelings is impossible. A dream is as real as life itself. If, say, the cast of *Glee* refused to allow her to join in a dance performance – as in last night's dream – then she is liable to feel rejected and sad all day. Clara has become particularly expert in the analysis of Melissa's dreams, trying to make sense of them and translating their experience from a negative to a positive.

At the same time as dealing with Melissa's problems, my MS was becoming ridiculous. I was getting oral steroids from my GP; I also had to self-inject Copaxone once a week and it triggered the most horrible flu-like symptoms for 24 hours plus a cracking headache. I was violently sick and couldn't cope with the light. Effectively, I lost 24 hours in every seven days and I was on it for a year. Andrew ended up having to do the injections until I came to the conclusion that the chances of it helping my MS were so remote that I'd rather not use it. I used to take it on a Friday night and lose half the weekend with my kids. Some people with MS will try anything: special oxygenated water, French remedies, Californian drugs … I know others who have bought drugs over the Internet. 'Snake Venom Blessed By Virgins at Dawn' syndrome is how I would describe this hopeful attitude.

I myself run everything past Dr Weller, my consultant at the Western General Hospital.

'What do you think?'

She always gives me an honest, thought-through response. When I was a health visitor, I used to tell my patients: 'Look, loads of people will give you advice: choose someone you trust and filter everything through them. Don't believe everything and don't take everything on.'

My other key support over the years was my physiotherapist Paula Cowan. She tried everything: I've had Botox in my calf muscles (ouch and no jokes about foreheads and wrinkles!), electrical stimulation, stretching exercises and drug therapy. Paula also listened – a lot – as I poured out my broken heart at not being able to walk properly. I had assumed the Botox would release the spasm to the point where I could run up a hill again; that was stupid. In fact, it only meant that I didn't drag my foot so far along the floor. That was deemed a success, but not for me.

Other than that, medically I was on my own: I was in secondary progressive. Once a year, I went to see my consultant, who said something along the lines of 'You're going downhill. I know I've promised you drug trials – you never fit the criteria. It might have to be a private prescription. There might be a new drug available in the next couple of years that might dampen the spasms, there might not.'

When I wake up in the morning I never know what part of me might not work – it's still like living with Damocles' sword hanging over your head. My old war wounds are getting worse. Up until this point I managed the steady deterioration of my body by dreaming up the next crazy scheme. In 2007, I learnt how to scuba dive – it was my way of managing the MS, a distraction. I found a local company who offered tuition, Deep Blue Scuba, and rang them up.

'Can you cope with someone who can't use her legs?' I asked.

With a brilliant woman called Beth, I began lessons in a swimming pool in Fettes. Predictably, I took longer than everyone else. I really struggled with my hands to do the valve connections, to attach and release my Bouyancy Compensator Device but Beth was determined I would succeed – and so I did. I passed the theory test, too. By the end of two full weekends I was deemed safe enough to do open dives in Loch Long. In PADI, you have to do two open-water dives and demonstrate all the skills learnt in the pool in 'open water' – I dived with webbed gloves to maximise strokes and stubby fins that weighed less than flippers.

It was as if the water had healing powers: the pain in my arms and legs literally vanished. I loved the independence, the sound of my breath, just bubbles and silent blue. In Loch Long it was so dark and murky, I couldn't see my hand in front of my face and had to do a walk-in entry. Beth was clear: we will help you to a point but you have to do all the skills yourself. At Dunbar we did a sea dive from the pier into fantastic, clear blue water. Did you know swimming through seaweed is like going through an underwater forest illuminated by shafts of sparkling sunlight?

That summer we went to Croatia so that I could dive in the crystal-clear waters of the Adriatic with its stunning fish. Everyone was so supportive and Andrew managed the children with his parents, who had come along to help. Yet faced with the climb out of the pool or the sea, I would feel the same overwhelming despair at the condition of my poor, painful body. Inevitably the change in temperature, the rush of cold air, would trigger a spasm and undo all the good work provided by the water.

I have a list of words that run through my mind whenever I'm feeling particularly despondent, words associated with MS:

Frustration   *Anger*
Fury   *Ghost (disappear)*

Night Falls

Pain   *Lost*
Grieving   *Fear*
Loss   *Desperation*
Useless

I could dive, but I could no longer swim; I'd go round and round in circles in the water, such was my life. I'd been given a wheelchair after suffering from tendonitis in my shoulder because of the pressure of using crutches. However, I could still walk and was therefore deemed mobile by the NHS, who refused to allocate me an electric wheelchair: this meant that I had no crutches, no Zimmer and no NHS wheelchair. When my aunt's father died, I inherited his little electric wheelchair. It was a real lifesaver: now I could still get out.

My physiotherapist told me that clients say there's a sense of relief when you get into the wheelchair. My answer to this would be relief and sadness, actually. The good news was I could go to the post-office, the hairdresser and the local newsagent to pick up my newspaper, unaided. Once there, I could get out of the shop again, unaided. I used the wheelchair for the first time to go to the cinema and suddenly the MS stopped being hidden: I had a piece of equipment and people were opening doors for me. The sad thing is that in my dreams I can walk and run; I am never in the chair. And so for a split second when I wake in the mornings, I have forgotten until the pain and spasms hit me.

I began to use the disabled parking space in Clara's old school. One day a teacher accused me, quite angrily, of misusing the space. When I told him I had MS, he replied: 'People like you shouldn't even have children!' That was kind.

The wheelchair brought its own frustrations, with which I struggle to this day. Public life wasn't designed for disabled people: the check-out counters are too high, making it impossible to give the cashier your purse; pavements are uneven (and sometimes disappear), there are no ramps, there isn't enough room between racks in department stores to access the clothes, thoughtless morons park in the disabled spaces on the premise of, *Oh I'm just popping in* … You see them jumping out of their Audis and running into the shop.

I can't run but I've driven all the way to the shopping centre for a treat with Clara and now I'm going to have to sit and wait for you to run out with your three tonnes of shopping. Usually, I confront these people with, 'I think you've forgotten to display your blue disc.' Worse still, they're using their old mum's disc.

In fact, driving was becoming increasingly difficult. Previously I had trouble with it in the normal way because I couldn't apply enough pressure on the brakes to stop. My leg shook and so I had started to use hand controls but because of the weight of the car, it was now uncomfortable to drive and so getting anywhere grew harder and harder. Also, I panicked about leaving the house alone and I worried about what might happen if I needed help. The fact is, if you drop your purse or get stuck and can't get up the kerb then you have to ask someone to help, you have to explain why and you are dependent on strangers. I hated feeling vulnerable and dependent; it only added to my suffocating sense of disempowerment. What's more, I loathed being pushed in the wheelchair and still do – I'm very intolerant of it.

But I did have a new kitchen. In the spring of 2007, we had the house remodelled to accommodate the eventuality of me being in a wheelchair. It was either that or move to a much bigger house but we liked our house and the neighbourhood. We didn't want to move and so we worked with an occupational therapist on the redesign. The downstairs was pushed out to add an extra master bedroom (mine and Andrew's) and en suite for us. Our kitchen was extended and we also added a new family bathroom and utility room. We went from being a five-bed, one-bathroom house to a six-bed, three-bathroom property, with one bedroom serving as an office.

The extension was designed for a wheelchair-user: doors were widened and we spent months on the kitchen design. Some of the surfaces are dropped, others the right height for able-bodied people to use. The hob is on a dropped surface with a lock in case Melissa decides to 'play'. We keep my teabags in with the mugs, in the cupboard underneath the kettle where I can reach them. I also had the cupboard cut away under the sink with a 'half' cupboard underneath it – that way, I can wheel under the sink but the pipes are enclosed. My oven has a slide-away door so I don't have to reach over it or keep to one side of a hot oven to get things out. It works for me as a wheelchair-user but it doesn't scream 'disabled'.

Finding Harmony

The front of the house was mono-blocked to eliminate uneven surfacing and get rid of the steps leading up to the front door. It was cleverly done and the ramp up to the front door is all but invisible. The contractors also transplanted the privet hedge and now I can virtually drive to the front door. For the first time in years I could also get into the back garden. We had a wooden deck built and ramps that take me on a smooth elegant catwalk all the way from the back door to the back of the garden. From there, I can get to the garage where my disabled scooter lives. Once again I'm able to sit in my own garden having a coffee.

'This is so unfair,' declared Peter. 'After all those years of wanting a skateboard ramp and you wouldn't build me one. Now you've built one and I don't skateboard any more!'

He had a point.

So there we were in Wales, with Melissa weeping and washing her hands over the wrong Seekers' CD while I was exhausted and distressed. I spoke to the community paediatrician, who promised to phone me when we returned to Edinburgh. The next day, Melissa and I caught the plane and were picked up from the airport by Andrew.

It was lovely to be home but as we cleared the table after tea, Clara and Peter retreated to their bedrooms and I heard doors close and music thudding through the ceiling; I realised how disconnected I felt from them. Peter and Clara were now teenagers and they needed their own space. It was a stage of life, a fact of life. Yet because I couldn't go bounding upstairs on the pretext of looking for dirty laundry or to find out what Peter was doing tomorrow, I didn't know what they were doing – or thinking. I felt doubly isolated from them.

I'd got to the stage where to wake them up in the morning I'd call their mobiles. I had my phone on me permanently, as did Peter and Clara. It was how we communicated inside and outside the house. I was also conscious of their need to escape the permanent scream-ing and distress downstairs: Mum wobbly in her wheel-chair and Melissa descending into panic and all the while me thinking, *we're losing her*.

The feelings of depression were scaring me and I knew being depressed was a far more disabling condition than the physical symptoms of MS. I didn't want to go back to that dark place, those woods, that fear and panic. The summer had taken its toll. Sensing the onset of depres-sion, I rang the social worker.

'I'm not coping,' I said. 'We're on our knees.'

The social worker for children affected by disability was hugely supportive but couldn't do much. The commu-nity paediatrician rang as promised and we were fast-tracked into a communication disorder clinic. Suddenly we had a condition, a passport to support: we went from zilch to something – at least it was more than before.

I remember Andrew sitting with me in the room in September 2008 and being told, very gently by the consultant, that Melissa was indeed on the autism spec-trum. *At last!* Neither of us was really surprised, more relieved there was now a label for our daughter's strange behaviour and fears. After I asked when the follow-up appointment would be, I was told there wouldn't be one.

OK, so we're on our own again.

Back home, I immediately went on the Internet and found both the National Autistic Society and the Lothian Autistic Society. The NAS had a superb course for parents/carers of newly diagnosed children; it was informative and helpful. There were so many things that made sense and so many suggestions to help. We used their befriending service and found a lovely young lady called Katy to help Melissa have fun. So, all of the work with Melissa is done by us or by friends, but knowledge helps, too.

Thanks to the social worker we were granted a few emergency respite hours during which Melissa would go off with an experienced autism worker. She loved it. I also valued the advice and help: I was taught some magic tricks to stem the panics and how to make timetables, time-lines and social stories to help Melissa manage her fear of uncertainty and the constant threat of chaos.

That summer we took Peter and Clara to a performance of capoeira from Brazil at the Fringe Festival. Afterwards, no one wanted to go home and so we went to a café for coffee and puddings. We all kept looking round as though part of us was missing.

'This makes a change,' observed Peter. 'We're actually going to *finish* a conversation?'

'But it's so quiet without Melissa,' said Clara.

All of us were wracked by the same conflict of emotions: on the one hand we missed Melissa, her constant questions and high-pitched chatter; on the other hand we were enjoying the opportunity to talk in a grown-up, conceptual way. We could leap from idea to idea without having to explain why blinded didn't literally mean to be blind, or pulling a leg wasn't physically pulling a leg. And we could talk in depth without dodging topics that might induce a panic. It was important for all of us to have that space although the next morning, I was very happy to see Melissa's beaming face once again.

10

Hope Dawns

September 2008. It was the first week of term, the beginning of a new school year and the house was empty. I had washed and dressed in my newly installed wet room; I'd reached the point where I needed grab rails, shower chairs and a long-handled, rubber-tipped brush (a bit like a scrubbing brush) which allowed me to wash my hair without having to keep my hands stretched above my head. The wet room gives me space and flexibility. I'd been very choosy about my grab rails: I didn't want boring functional stainless steel, I wanted cornflower blue – and I got them.

I got dressed apart from my socks (I can't put socks on myself and so as usual, I had cold feet). That day, I was wearing elasticated trousers and a baggy top. My core muscles have been shot to pieces and so trying to sit upright and hold my tummy in to look slim is now useless. These days I wear what's most comfortable for my body although I do try to avoid wearing tracksuits everyday. Tracksuits aren't good for self-esteem nor are fashion magazines. I hate fashion magazines – they conspire to make women feel fat and inadequate but I don't have time to explain why articles on 'Goodbye to Cellulite' are irrelevant when I've got that cotton-wool feeling in the side of my face.

For a long time I thought that I didn't deserve nice clothes until one day when a teenaged Clara asked: 'Mum, can I look in your wardrobe to borrow something to wear to the party on Saturday night?'

Little by little Clara took on the role of my personal stylist and shopper. She started going through my wardrobe and finding things for me to wear (as well as for herself!). I'm always convinced they won't fit me but when they do, I feel so good. Clara has worked really hard to reawaken the sense of fun I used to have with clothes. We've had a hilarious time trying to get high heels to work with a wheelchair (they don't, but it was fun trying). Most days I hate the way I look, but I'm happiest when Clara has dressed me. When I look at my daughter, I'm reminded that she's no longer my little baby (well, she *is*, and always will be). What I mean to say is, she's no longer the child she was. Clara loves fashion: she owns 36 pairs of shoes. She's growing up fast and I love watching the way she puts things together and looks so slim and beautiful. These days, if I have something to attend, I'll ask Clara to find an outfit and do my hair.

But back to reality: it was 10am on a Monday morning. Though sockless, I was otherwise dressed and already exhausted. I got myself to the kitchen, where I fed the rabbits (Duchess and Snuffles) and talked to the au pair about defrosting chicken legs and making a tomato sauce. Already I'd had to advise her on which temperature to set the washing machine in order to get rid of Peter's muddy rugby stains. Have you ever noticed how when your laundry is done by someone else, it's not so good as if you did it yourself? Likewise, it irritates me the way the clothes are hung – they're never hung properly. It's just a silly thing really, but when you can't do something your-self it's so incredibly frustrating – and you can't complain about the way they do it because you yourself can't do it at all.

As soon as I was able to do so, I escaped to my study. Some days my mind is like porridge. Imagine waking from a deep sleep or worse still, waking up after four hours of sleep and trying to get your brain in gear then imagine feeling like that everyday – that's how the MS feels. But it's no excuse not to do something and in this case, that something was to look for help and so I fired up the computer.

Gazing up at the framed photos on the wall of us on Everest, I thought about the fatigue I'd experienced, having walked seven kilometres to Base Camp as the clouds came in. I considered the pleasure of pain when you've reached the top of the mountain: your legs are quivering like jelly and your rucksack feels as if some-one's stuffed it with rocks; you can't speak with exhaus-tion. I thought of all the difficulties we had overcome to get there too. My most severe complaint had been blis-tered feet and a craving for a cup of strong PG Tips and some crunchy white bread and butter. That sort of pain is satisfying, unlike the daily grind of being unable to complete simple tasks.

My MS was becoming my new Everest, but it was an Everest I had come to dread. I dropped the pen. Well, it would have to stay there until Clara came home from school and picked it up! I hated being dependent on her. My thoughts turned back to the day ahead and the computer screen. What sort of extra support could I buy in? We already had our au pair. What else might I purchase? I studied various agency websites and their exorbitant costs – we couldn't afford them.

But then I googled 'disabled assistants Scotland'. Two words popped up on the screen: '*Canine Partners*'. I clicked on.

Assisting people with disabilities to enjoy greater independence and a greater quality of life.

'Independence' – the word jumped out at me. And so I read on. Two minutes later (in fact, probably less), I picked up the phone and rang the number on the screen. I had to know right there and then if I was the sort of person who would qualify for a Canine Partner. Curiously, I felt excited, so incredibly excited – it was a feeling I hadn't had for a long time. I was also nervous. What would they think? What would they say?

'Hello, Canine Partners.'

A lady called Julie picked up the phone. She was based down at Canine Partners' headquarters in Heyshott, West Sussex.

'Oh hello. My name's Sally and I was just reading about your charity on the Internet and wondering if it's true that you cover Scotland?' I asked.

'Yes,' she confirmed that they had indeed started to place dogs in Scotland.

We had a long chat and I explained my predicament: about my MS and Melissa's autism.

'We don't do joint partnerships – it would have to be your partnership,' Julie told me.

'That's absolutely fine,' I said. 'I understand completely.'

After all, if I had a dog to help me – a concept I still didn't fully understand – then surely I would have the energy to help Melissa too?

Julie warned me that there was a very long waiting list. However, the good news was that Scottish Canine Partners had just been set up and so I could qualify. Trembling with anticipation, I thanked her and put down the phone. Was this what I'd been looking for? Could it be the answer to my prayers?

Two days later, as promised, I received an application pack. As soon as I'd got the kids off to school, I sat down and began filling in the form: *Name. Address. Mobility levels. Main reasons for wanting a Canine Partner.* I paused and took a deep breath: I had to be painfully, brutally honest about my needs and expectations here. This was it – I had nothing to lose and everything to gain. And so I began writing.

Being asked to give ways that a canine companion could help me is like being in a restaurant and being asked to order anything you want!

DAILY ROUTINE
- *Perhaps a dog could go upstairs and wake up the children? Certainly I would like to think he/she could go and get Peter and Clara in an emergency, i.e. if I fell.*
- *Assistance with picking up shoes and socks in the morning and giving them to me. I find getting anything from the floor very difficult.*
- *After the school run, I go and pick up my newspaper. The newspaper shop has a step and I usually have to wait for someone to go in and collect my newspaper for me. It would be great if a dog could go in and do this for me.*
- *In my office, there are many ways a dog could help me. I struggle with retrieving files, picking up things from the floor (I always miss the waste paper basket!).*
- *When I prepare dinner (with au pair), could the dog open drawers and cupboards for me?*
- *By the evening I am so tired and sore that I am constantly dropping things and need to collect things to help with the children's homework. Perhaps the dog could help with this?*

OCCASIONAL
- *Wednesdays, I take Melissa to her swimming lessons. I can definitely see how an assistance dog could help me to be a 'proper mum' by getting the clothes out of the*

swimming bag so that I can change Melissa from a
sitting position.

- *Library: The library has introduced a new automated
  service, which I find incredibly difficult. I go every
  week and it would be superb if a dog could help me
  with putting books into slots, etc.*
- *Extra shopping: The dog can perhaps help with my
  purse and putting things into my bag?*
- *Cinema/theatre, etc: I find juggling tickets, wheelchair,
  programme too much. Could a dog assist?*

WEEKEND
- *(Husband home/Lie-in/Husband does weekly shop)*
- *Attend church: I would feel much less 'disabled' if I
  had a dog to collect hymnbooks, etc.*

OTHER THINGS A DOG MIGHT BE ABLE TO DO
- *Use the cashpoint machine.*
- *Could a dog assist me with stretching in some way? I
  find if someone puts weights on my leg then it assists
  the pain of the spasms.*
- *'Tell' someone who has rung the bell that I'm on my
  way. I often get to the door to find that the person has
  gone.*
- *I never seem to be where the phone is, so to have it
  brought to me would be grand. I often find myself
  transferred into my chair and then realise I don't have
  the remote control or phone, or some other essential
  device. Could a dog do it, rather than my bellowing for
  Clara to come and do it?*

- *Alert someone if I have a problem.*
- *On bad days when my arm is useless, press the button at the zebra crossing for me.*

PERSONAL STATEMENT
I would love to have a Canine Partner. I feel as if I am constantly relying on the goodwill of others, particularly my husband and children. My condition fluctuates but my current 'baseline' is poor. My world has become very small and each outing requires so much energy trying to overcome obstacles. I would dearly love my kids to be kids, and me to be a fully functioning member of the world again!

Phew! Was that asking too much? Would a furry, four-legged, canine friend really be able to provide such a level of care and commitment? Wouldn't he rather chase foxes (we have a family of fearless foxes living behind our shed) and run after sticks? I was asking a dog to give me back my life; it was preposterous yet seemingly possible. At the same time I realised I wanted it *so* badly.

The next section of the form asked the applicant to confirm their willingness and ability to exercise a dog for one hour each day. I was impressed that the dog's best interests were given top priority but as I would soon discover, the dog's needs are at the heart of the Canine Partners' philosophy: your disability is invisible, it's all about the dog.

I hid the application letters, leaflets and magazines in my underwear drawer so that no one, apart from Andrew, knew. I didn't want them to be disappointed or sceptical at this stage. It was my little nugget of fun.

Once I'd sent off my initial application, I didn't have to wait long before I received the next enormous bunch of forms. This time I had to fill in details about my family and me. I gave Canine Partners permission to consult my GP, my occupational therapist and my MS consultant and then I had to sign a release form. All the Scottish medical professionals I use were brilliantly efficient in sending back the right documents. My wonderful occupational therapist even faxed them a huge assessment document stating that I *really* needed a dog. The comments at Heyshott were: 'Gosh, things do move quickly in Scotland!'

Obviously I then had to let family and friends know about my secret plan. We didn't tell Melissa at this stage because she would have assumed that we meant it would be happening immediately. Perhaps not surprisingly, most people (other than Andrew) queried the wisdom of my decision.

'How can you look after a dog?'

'Are you sure you can look after a dog?'

And even: 'Do you really think it's a good idea to take on the responsibility of a dog as well as everything else?'

Doubts began to set in. You only have to think of dog hero Marley in the hilarious memoir *Marley & Me* grabbing the lead and shaking his head from side to side or taking off after a cat. What if he or she spied a bunch of four-legged friends on the other side of the park and bolted off, leaving me with a tangled lead? I wouldn't be able to control a crazy puppy. Or what if the dog suddenly lunged forward and dragged me out of my wheelchair?

Overriding all of the above concerns was the very simple question of how I'd clean up after a dog. OK, so now I was really worried. I rang Canine Partners.

'What about picking up poo?' I asked.

'Don't worry,' said Julie. 'We have systems and ways to teach you how to look after your dog. There are commands for everything. If you were to get a dog, you would learn commands. We would teach you all you need to know about how to care for your dog in the best way for you.'

'What about exercising?' I persisted.

But she just laughed: 'Yes, we have that sorted too.'

11

Starting a New Adventure

I sent off the final batch of forms and crossed my fingers. Now that I had a plan it was as though someone had shown me a secret door. Already it was partly open and through it I'd caught a glimpse of a sunny day and a beautiful Golden Labrador chasing a ball. When, a week later, I received a letter offering me an applicant assessment day in November 2008, the door was yanked open wide: now I could see the sky.

But before I got there, I had a list of commands to learn:

'Come here!'	*'Sit!/Down!/Stand!'*
'Behind!'	*'Heel!/Side!'*
'Let's go!'	*'Better go now!'*
'Get it!'	*'Bring it here!'*
'My lap!'	*'Knee!'*

The big day came and when I say big, I mean BIG. I was so excited, I couldn't talk and a silent Sally makes everyone nervous. The family were giving me very strange looks.

'Mum, are you all right?'

'Fine, fine,' I insisted.

How would it go? Would I return disappointed, deemed unable to care for a dog or would I be able to master the lessons and ... I just couldn't handle the idea of failure.

Andrew and I flew down from Edinburgh to Gatwick and hired a car. We were doing it as a day trip to reduce the amount of time that he took off (he was now working in London on a consultancy basis) and we left Melissa behind. The team provided by Gatwick to collect me from the plane were a bit confused and dropped us off at International Arrivals. Quite why we were taken to International Arrivals, we still don't know. It might have been funny, being asked for my passport, if time hadn't been of the essence.

'Sorry,' I said. 'I didn't think we needed passports travelling from Scotland.'

Eventually they let us through but we still had to get past Customs.

We arrived at Gatwick to one of those glorious cold autumnal days. We drove past thick woods. Leaves shimmered in a patchwork of orange and gold, then the landscape opened out and we arrived at Heyshott – a small village with a church and a nature reserve, where they've discovered Neolithic and Bronze Age earthworks. We turned left into the long, sweeping drive through fields on either side. As we did so, we passed a sign:

SLOW 10 MPH
Wheelchairs and dogs in all parts of the site

We were definitely in the right place! After turning right into the complex of buildings, we parked up. On the left was what turned out to be the newly built residential units in what was once a stable block; they looked like pretty cottages. I found out later that their chief volunteer gardener (William) had made sure there were tubs of colour, even in November. To give you a little bit of background, Canine Partners has been there since 2003, when the charity was able to buy a former polo yard and farm with various outbuildings. The polo tack room had been converted into a training room.

It was 10.30am by the time we entered the big converted barn that serves as Canine Partners headquarters and I was definitely frazzled. I'd phoned to apologise in advance for my lateness but felt frantic with anxiety; it wasn't a good start. In fact it turned out that Chrissie, the trainer whose job it was to assess me, was late too, which made me feel a whole lot better. Later, I discovered that they were quite accustomed to people being subject to the vagaries of public transport.

The barn was empty: we found ourselves in a big reception area, looking up at a balcony that runs all the way around the top. We weren't sure what to do. In a room to the left we could glimpse people in purple, dogs and someone in a wheelchair. We waited, eventually knocked and were welcomed with a smile: 'Hello! You must be Sally, I'm Chrissie,' plus the offer of a cup of tea and then ushered into the next-door room.

Chrissie was very friendly and welcoming; she asked me about the journey and explained how the day would run. First, we would get to know each other a bit and have a chat. Then we would meet the dogs, have lunch, do some work with the dogs and then a final chat. Unable to think straight, I was so scared and nervous that I just kept nodding. I was transported back to the church halls of my nursing days when I was involved in running children's drama groups and listening to them belting out their lines while giving lots of encouragement.

'*Stop! Who goes there?*'

Instead of being draughty and smelling of dust, however, the place was warm, light and wonderfully peaceful. The only interruptions to the library-like quiet were occasional barks from the dogs. There were dogs everywhere: they were all on vets' beds (they have a special kind of bed fabric for dogs), some lying, others barking, still more sitting. Some were in advanced training, others staying there while their partners were in hospital and some were even being re-partnered. I was amazed at how quiet the site was, given the number of dogs – it was a far cry from Battersea Dogs & Cats Home or the local vet. If you hadn't seen all those dogs on site, you might have thought they were all out for the day.

Two other people were being assessed that day: both female, one younger, one much older than me, but both in wheelchairs. We didn't really make contact other than smiling as we were all focused on this new experience. It did, however, make me feel better that I wasn't the only newbie.

'Just ignore the dogs,' said Chrissie. 'They're here to work and we have our own reward system.'

I'd been wondering what they used as secret weapons.

We went through the form so that Andrew and I could ask questions. I felt that I should ask a few to show interest but I was so tongue-tied (a phenomenon that rarely happens to me) that I was grateful for Andrew's useful questions about caring for the dogs and our set-up at home. I felt like a little kid: I just wanted to meet the dogs. *Show me the dogs!* I could feel myself becoming more and more impatient; I tried to behave: *Don't be stroppy, Sally!* I could feel Andrew looking at me, trying to keep me calm.

'So,' said Chrissie, getting up. 'Shall we meet the dogs?'

At last! The first Golden Labrador I met was Garfield, an apt name for the floppy-haired, burnt-toffee dog. He was brought to me and attached to my wheelchair using the cunning fixtures and clever leads devised by Canine Partners as part of their system. All the dogs that I would meet that day were in advanced training; already they had been partnered or were about to be partnered and so they knew what they were doing. They were ideal dogs for me to work with while being assessed.

An electric wheelchair was produced and I was shown how to use it: another first. When I say first, I mean this was the first time I'd willingly used an electric wheelchair beyond the four walls of my home. On bad days when my legs were shaky, I used the little one at home. It felt strange but at the same time, a positive experience. But Canine Partners make no fuss over your disabilities: the focus is on the dog, and how you and the dog can work as a team.

I was then shown how the special Canine Partners' lead works. It's a brilliant design: 1.2 metres (4 feet) long, with metal rings at intervals that can be attached to the wheelchair via a connection on the chair. The lead is let out at intervals by taking rings on and off, giving the dog length, according to what you need it to do. Say, for example, you need the dog to go behind your chair when you're going through a door then you must let them have a full length.

I was so concerned with trying to negotiate the dog and the lead while remembering my commands at the same time that I kept forgetting to turn the wheelchair off whenever I stopped.

'Wheelchair off!' said Chrissie.

It was both humbling and frustrating to forget such a simple task; it was much harder than anticipated too. The coordination necessary to move in a wheelchair with a dog involves a feat of logic – it's a marriage of minds and machinery. If you're turning left, you say 'move!' – the dogs are trained to move out of the way. When turning right, however, you say nothing. You always start with 'Let's go!' so the dog knows you are on the move.

Was it easy to confuse? You bet! Yet suddenly being in a wheelchair felt like more of an advantage than a disadvantage: now I was able to move easily round a room with a gorgeous dog in tow, looking at me and listening to me. I was in control of my life. Thrilled, I kept glancing over at Andrew (a huge animal-lover), knowing how much he wanted to go over to the dogs who weren't working and give them a stroke. He was so fantastic, though and didn't make eye contact with them at all. It must have been pretty dull for him to just sit and watch.

But Andrew can handle pressure well: occasionally he would catch my eye with a silent 'go on, you can do this!'. I wanted to get it right for my sake, for his sake and for our kids. Most of all, I was keen to prove that I could master the exercises for the sake of Garfield, who was beginning to look confused: *Are you turning right or left, lady? Make your mind up!*

Chrissie then asked me to drop some keys and a purse on the floor, which I duly did.

'Get it, bring it here!' I said, as I became more accustomed to the manoeuvring.

Then I got the commands wrong and poor Garfield did nothing. When he should have retrieved, I told him, 'Bring it here!' bypassing the 'Get it!' altogether. Now I was in a real fluster.

'I think we all need a cup of tea,' said Chrissie, just in the nick of time.

Half an hour later I was back with the dogs. This time I was passed on to a black Flat-coat called Guy. Flat-coats are manic: often they are called 'Peter Pan dogs' because they remain eternally youthful and playful. Guy's tail flapped, his ears flapped and his tongue hung out as though he'd already run a marathon and was eager to do another. I remember thinking, *how am I going to control this dog?* I could hear my voice rising; he was making me nervous. As we went around the room retrieving items and opening doors, I was feeling tense.

Afterwards I said it was like trying to control a thoroughbred stallion. I thought he was the most amazing dog in the world but in retrospect, he didn't make me feel safe. He ended up being partnered with a man and apparently they're both very happy, which is brilliant. I've always had a soft spot for Guy and follow his adventures. One posting on Facebook by his partner recently read: 'If anyone in Holland sees a flat-coat swimming by, could you tell him his tea's ready!' It made me laugh. He's a lovely dog, but too much for me.

We'd brought a picnic lunch, which we ate in the other room with my fellow applicants. Though tired, everyone chatted about where they had come from and what they hoped for from the dogs. I hardly ate or spoke, which again wasn't like me at all.

Afterwards we had coffee before putting on outdoor clothes and going out to the backfield to exercise the dogs. Again, that's not as easy as it sounds. First, we had to negotiate getting out there, which involved going through a door, passing between a row of parked cars and bringing the dogs with us. I managed it and what's more, Garfield didn't get tangled up with me.

We then had to take the dogs to the toilet area and tell them to use it with a 'Better go now!' instruction, then wait. *Aha, so that's how you pick up poo!* I thought. In fact, you don't. Instead the dog goes in a special toilet area so that it doesn't need to relieve itself in a public place. They learn to control their bowels and go when instructed – very clever.

The field was surrounded by hedges, the air fresh and cold: it was exactly what I needed to wake me from the stupor brought on by a 5am start, intense concentration and a warm room. The ground was bumpy. Being outside was turning into an off-road adventure.

'I'm going to show you the first task you need,' said Chrissie, 'which is a controlled release of the lead. You let the dog off the lead, you count to ten then say, "Release. Go play!" Got it?'

'I think so,' I said.

We had a few practice sessions. I'd forgotten what it was to feel a sense of achievement at having mastered a new skill: I felt responsible for the dog and I loved it, all of it. To share his freedom, to know he would respond to whatever I said felt amazing. It was also fantastic to be outside playing with this animal. Memories of running across fields with Shep, watching Jet scamper across the South Downs or seeing Sandie hurl her barrel-shaped body into the sea came flooding back.

I raced all round the little field in my wheelchair. Chrissie only intervened once when I was chasing Garfield.

'We don't encourage the dogs to run away from the person in the chair,' she told me. 'Otherwise, when you need them they might think it's a game.'

With Andrew by my side, I worked with lots of different dogs. I had to get them to retrieve their toys and bring them back to me. Chrissie stood and watched, looking cold and chatting with other trainers who were bringing dogs over to the toilet areas. Afterwards she smiled and said, 'Well done!'

But did she mean it? I was absolutely exhausted but too scared to ask if I could have a dog. Meanwhile, the trainers had lunch and discussed applicants as Andrew and I took a much-needed cup of tea.

'It's so difficult standing around all those dogs and not being able to stroke them,' said Andrew.

I couldn't have agreed more. Andrew is the St Francis in our family. Dogs just love him, as do cats, horses and well, just about any animal you care to mention, really – his calm persona attracts them. Chrissie left us alone for a while and Andrew sneaked a quick stroke with Guy.

After lunch, we waited for Chrissie at the table in the barn and I tried to pretend my stomach really wasn't twisted into knots or that my entire future was predicated on whether or not I was suitable for a Canine Partnership.

Chrissie came and sat down opposite us.

'Yes,' she said.

Yes?

'We do think you're suitable for a dog. Now, what else do you want the dog to do?'

I couldn't believe it: I'd passed the first hurdle and I was overjoyed.

Andrew squeezed my hand.

'Thanks, Chrissie,' I said.

On the plane home that evening I was so exhausted and in so much pain that I couldn't sleep. I just kept thinking, *I'm going to get a dog; I'm going to get a dog!*

12

Love at Second Sight

In retrospect, perhaps we shouldn't have tried to fit it all in a single day: meeting the dogs, learning about Canine Partners, them learning about me. When I got on the plane, I was aching from head to toe but of course, I couldn't sleep: I was buzzing with excitement. It was like the first flush of love when you can't stop giggling but you're racked with anxiety, all at the same time. I shut my eyes and revisited the experience: the smells of the dogs, the fresh air, the beauty of the countryside and the slow dawning realisation that this was to be my new adventure.

Was it going to work out?

We got home after dark and went straight to bed. In the morning, with Andrew off to work I talked to Melissa about our day over the snap, crackle and pop of her Rice Krispies. She thought we had been to a meeting (in some ways, it is a benefit of her disability that she doesn't ask too many questions). Then she was off to school and didn't seem to think any more about it. Keeping our plans for a dog a secret from her was so difficult.

But the older kids knew where I was going: I had kept the leaflets well hidden but I couldn't resist telling them all about it. Although they didn't quite grasp the assistance bit, they were hugely excited about the prospect of getting a dog; they had also taken on board the 'hands off' approach – a difficult one to instil when you have a family.

Meanwhile, I kept reading the first leaflet I had been sent and the stories of disabled people who have Canine Partners. Gazing at their photos, I wondered if I would be like them one day. The leaflet had become a lucky charm. In retrospect, I'd already sensed the dark clouds lifting, as if the very thought of another adventure for Andrew and me was beginning to work its magic.

Two weeks later I had a call from Canine Partners to say that they wanted to do a home visit to make sure ours was suitable. In the first week of December 2008, partnership coordinator Wendy and Adele (PA to Andy Cook, the chief executive) travelled up from Heyshott to look round and meet the family.

As I have already mentioned, our house is detached. From the kitchen, French doors open directly out onto wooden decking, from which a series of ramps access the garden. Taking Adele and Wendy for a tour, Andrew explained we would organise the toilet area to the left of the ramp, not too far away from the house, which would make it more pleasant if the weather was bad; it would also be well away from the garden shed, where the foxes live. They asked us to install gates on either side of the house to block the two points of access from front to back. Ironically, my final comment was that a blonde dog wouldn't be good because I've got purple carpets.

Wendy and Adele signed me off. I'd passed the second hurdle! The next couple of weeks flew by in a flurry of activities. Clara was in her last year in the choir and was one of the head choristers. This meant shouldering solos, organisational duties and also being present at rehearsals, concerts and services. Since she had been in the choir, Christmas Eve and Christmas Day had tight schedules of their own. Clara would do the second of two Nine Lessons and carols (the traditional service leading up to Christmas and my favourite because it's always so mysterious and magical). The choir begins in the pitch-black with the 'Once in Royal David's City' solo and then launches into a series of carols, lighting candles as they proceed into the cathedral. That year, Clara and the other head chorister rotated the solo with 'In the Bleak Midwinter'. It was such a proud moment hearing my daughter's voice soar, not for the first time, into the rafters.

On Christmas Eve Clara would finish at 9pm, come home for a bowl of soup and have to be back by 10.30pm for a rehearsal before the Midnight Service and communion (Andrew always attended this). While they were away, I would wrap presents and put them in the stockings. We still do this, even though Melissa is the only one who believes in the existence of the generous, bearded gentleman from the North Pole. Bleary-eyed, Clara and Andrew would stumble home at about 1am. By then Melissa had already put out the whisky, shortbread and a carrot for Rudolph.

Having got into bed at about 1.30am, Clara had to be awake and in the cathedral again for the morning service, which meant a 9.30am rehearsal. We still managed to open the stockings beforehand but saved the big presents until after the service when we would drive for 10 minutes to Murrayfield to spend the day with my in-laws. I'm really proud of my children and their attitude to Christmas: let's eke it out for as long as we can! Often we are still opening gifts on Boxing Day and the day after, enjoying each present before moving onto the next. One year, the first one when we did the 'shoeboxes' – a charitable act whereby you fill a shoebox with as many things as you can and wrap it in brightly coloured paper for the less fortunate – Peter said: 'Before we open our presents, can we think about the boys and girls who are only getting shoeboxes and the ones who aren't even getting that.' I'm so proud of my kids' awareness of others.

Meanwhile, I kept hoping, waiting for the post and doing my best to contain the excitement; I was like a big kid again. All Christmas, the same thoughts were going round and round my head:

Could my new dog really reshape our lives? Were we asking too much?

I was told that Canine Partners were waiting for a new batch of dogs in January. The dogs were currently living with families. Part of Canine Partners' system is to find and train up teams of so-called 'puppy parents' (canine foster parents, if you like) who rear the puppies for their first, very important year but then have the heartbreak of handing them back. Those puppies deemed suitable then go on to advanced training in what I dubbed 'boarding school' – the kennels at the headquarters in Heyshott.

I knew the waiting list was long and there was no guarantee any of the dogs would be suitable, but it didn't stop me from hoping. Christmas passed in its usual blur of activities and fun, complete with overexcited and exhausted children. Boxing Day was always a good excuse to wrap up warm and take everyone out for a walk. Sometimes we would go to Cramond and Silvernowes, with its glorious esplanade, perfect for learning to ride bikes. Always there are lots of eager kids wobbling along on shiny new bikes on 26 December. The week between Christmas and Hogmanay was spent making sure the children's thank you letters were written: even before they could write, I would make them draw something to send as a thank-you.

In January 2009 I received the Christmas present I'd been hoping for: a letter from Canine Partners inviting me to attend a two-day assessment programme the same month. I couldn't believe my luck. When I rang Mum to tell her the good news, she was adamant that she wanted to come with me (Andrew couldn't get the time off work and she was dying to see what it was all about). With only two weeks' notice, there was a lot to organise: we flew down to Gatwick, hired a car and drove to Heyshott. That sounds simpler than it was. In fact, it was an impressive feat for Mum, who had to manage a new car plus busy roads and motorways (latterly, all she had driven on were island and Scottish highland roads), but she drove brilliantly.

Mum and I would be staying in the fantastic, newly built residential unit. A team of occupational therapists had been consulted on the design, which means every aspect of living with a disability had been considered. There are six purpose-built chalets with wet rooms; one has a bath for pain relief. All have overhead hoists so you can be hoisted from your bed to a wheelchair, and from a wheelchair to the loo, if necessary. There are profiling beds (beds that can rise up and down for comfort, like the ones in hospitals) and all sorts of gadgets to make life easier: switches, alarm buttons and touch-sensor bedside lamps. Everything is adapted for maximum comfort.

Canine Partners match a person to a chalet according to their need for a bath or shower, a close-mat toilet (the wash-and-blowdry of the toilet world) and if they need extra room for another bed. Grab rails are everywhere and hoists available, if necessary. Wonderful! Even the kitchen and dining room were designed by a wheelchair-user, which means there are specially adapted fridges, freezers and hobs, all at the perfect height. Everything has been thought through, with no compromises – it's the equivalent of staying in a five-star hotel. What's more, we were among the first to stay there, which made the experience doubly special.

The Canine Partners' philosophy is to make wheelchair-users feel as comfortable as possible so they can concentrate on working with the dogs, and that's exactly what happened with me. In addition to a trainer, everyone has a carer allocated, if they require it. The carers stay on site to help with whatever makes everyday life easier for those with disabilities and their dogs while they train.

This time around my trainer was a woman called Claire. She was a tall, willowy girl, with a great sense of humour and in common with all the other trainers that I met she was also a calm, patient person. After the format of the day had been explained to us and Mum set off on a trip to meet a friend in Chichester, Claire brought a dog out for me to meet. This was to be the way it worked: meet a dog and work with them, then that dog would go away and you would meet another one, do some more work and so on.

'Today, we need to do some of the more difficult tasks,' she told us.

The new batch of dogs included Elmo, Headley, Foster and Harmony: three males and a female. There was also Harry and Henry, two Golden Retrievers who I always confused. Elmo, a Retriever Labrador Cross with a golden coat and huge brown eyes, needed a new home (his previous partner was now too ill to manage a Canine Partner). He was very calm and exuded an 'I know what I'm doing' air. I liked him immediately and this time around, I felt more relaxed with the place and its routines.

Then I was given Foster to work with. Foster was a lovely Golden Retriever who wasn't coping with 'boarding school' and so was being fostered by a family and attending 'day school'. The move to accommodate Foster's needs is just another example of how well Canine Partners care for each dog as individuals. The dog's mental and physical wellbeing is of paramount importance.

We did picking up, retrieval and the supermarket checkout sequence. As usual I got into a real muddle but Claire just smiled, told funny stories and helped me focus. Again, it seemed ridiculously complicated and I kept on muddling the length of the lead, but the dogs usually managed to avoid getting in a tangle and the trainers were brilliant, too. The next day Mum was watching from the balcony (no pressure there, then!) but that also made me feel proud for she was witnessing something new and exciting.

At lunch, Claire asked: 'Do you have a preference?'

'Elmo and Headley at number one, with Harmony and Harry close seconds,' I said.

'Why?'

I thought for a moment, then said: 'Harmony was too quiet for me – she seemed very passive. I loved Elmo's confidence and I liked the way Headley looked at me so much.'

We talked a bit more about my life thus far, my lifestyle, the kids, my work and what exactly I'd need the dog to do. I told her about Sandie and Shep, and Jet too. Although I was able to ask lots of questions, I was almost too scared to do so in case I talked myself out of getting a dog. I didn't want to blame any of the dogs for not responding to me in case I was blotting my own copybook and I could see how the trainers were trying to marry the practical aspects of my life with a good personality match but I had no idea how they did this. As I was to realise later, they do it with great success. Claire's observation of my interaction with the dogs was useful for me too. She gave me feedback on how to talk to them and also commented that I seemed too quiet with the dogs: *Quiet, moi?*

'They are all just so amazing,' I said. 'I'm scared to do something wrong – they are such special dogs!'

'Remember, they are just dogs not angels,' she told me gently.

'I'll remember that,' I said.

As the day progressed, I spent time with other dogs and became more adept at knowing which ones I found good to work with and those I didn't find quite so easy. Then I put on my coat and went outside with Foster and Vicky, another trainer. For a while, I played with Foster – throwing balls, rehearsing commands – but I found him unresponsive. I had to work hard to get him to do stuff with me; he didn't seem to look at me much. In retrospect, this was exactly what Vicky was there to pick up on. What sort of chemistry did we have? On the way back, I apologised for how tricky it had been with Foster.

'It's fine,' she insisted. 'You did well because you didn't throw all your toys out of the pram and you persisted with him. That's good!'

Phew, another hurdle overcome and I needed all the praise I could get. Proof indeed that humans and dogs have to click, just like people.

'Do you know who this is?' asked Becca, the head trainer.

'Harmony,' I replied.

Already Harmony seemed to have more bounce and spring in her step than Foster. She gave me a huge cuddle, which made me laugh. Was I really that special or did she flirt outrageously with everyone she met? Becca left us while Vicky stayed to watch.

It was a frosty afternoon. You could hear the wood pigeons cooing and see the church spire silhouetted against a pale sky. I was transported back to afternoons as a little girl, playing with the dogs and rolling around on the grass. When I was small I could wrap my arms around Sandie's neck until she shook her head and I'd tumble backwards like a sack of potatoes. Sandie and Shep had been my playmates, Jet was my companion and now I was looking for a companion and friend but also a dog that could help me: the term 'assistance dog' made sense.

It's easy to find common ground with younger dogs if you have a ball. I threw the ball for Harmony and watched her decide *not* to pick it up. Instead she chose to inspect every single blade of grass by the hedge and then leapt into the air as if she had just discovered the spring in her step.

Hey, look at this – I've got a tail! And I can jump in circles.

Despite earlier reservations, I found myself entranced and hugely entertained. The smells of the countryside seemed to unlock a hidden part of Harmony and release her curiosity. All of a sudden she was the funniest, friendliest dog you could ever hope to meet. I didn't mind her slinking off: her need for solitude was evidence of a desire to understand the world. Indeed I respected her desire for a quiet moment all the more when she wheeled round and bounded over for a cuddle.

When I told her to 'Get it!' and 'Bring it here!' in order to retrieve the ball, she did as she was told and we had a great time playing ball and running together, her on four legs and me on four wheels. The wind in my hair was a magical part of life that I'd missed – until now.

By end of the day, I was exhausted and no one was giving anything away. I just knew that one day I would get a dog. Meanwhile, the trainers were saying things like, '*If* we match you this time,' and, '*If* there's no match this time you can keep coming until we find a match.' I was also exhilarated. Mum says there was a change in my voice whenever I mentioned Harmony; I wasn't aware of this at the time and I don't remember it, but she says she knew that I was keen on Harmony, which speaks volumes about a mother's intuition.

That night over a delicious supper of lasagne and salad prepared by Shirley, the doyenne of housekeepers, we chatted about the day. The on-duty trainers were there, as were the dogs; some were the trainer's dogs and others were dogs-in-training. We ate in a small room with tables barely large enough to accommodate us all. It wasn't the most peaceful of meals but certainly one of the happiest. I met a lady called Claire with her dog Ulli: she is a trustee who was there for a meeting. Claire and Ulli were long-term partners and I was amazed by their seamless relationship. I watched in awe for Ulli seemed to instinctively know what Claire wanted and needed – I was so envious of their teamwork.

It was also the first time that I discovered the secret of the cream cheese tubes. The reward system is based on high and low rewards: bits of carrot and broccoli are low, while cream cheese is high (and no, I'd never thought of giving a dog cream cheese either!). The advantage of the cream cheese tube is that it's transportable and you don't have to put your hand into a wet mush of carrot, sausage, broccoli and cheese mix while travelling. Instead you roll up the tube and let the dog lick a bit from the end.

I asked Claire lots of questions: in fact, I grilled her. How much does Ulli do for you? Does she get enough exercise? Do you ever worry that she might be bored? Does it feel like an awfully big responsibility caring for a dog? She gave me so much encouragement and advice that I left our conversation feeling reassured and able to imagine life with a dog – it was a fantastic boost at this stage in the process.

We also met a dog who was back at Canine Partners with a view to being given a new partner: a young black Labrador, who my mother instantly fell in love with and wanted to take home. He would be going to a new partner but Mum knew that Canine Partners hold a waiting list of good, vetted homes for those dogs no longer able to assist a disabled person. In the end her head won over her heart and she decided not to ask for details of the dog.

I slept well that night aware that Mum was in the room next door in case I needed her. The next morning I woke to the knowledge that I would be going home and wondered if there would be a dog for me. Or had I already met him or her? Breakfast was a jolly affair and a welcome coffee got me going. I was beginning to sense the MS 'porridge' effect creeping in but I knew I could beat it: I had dogs to meet.

After breakfast I was introduced to Ann, my trainer for the day. Apparently if Canine Partners think they are drawing close to a match then that dog's trainer works with the potential partnership, but I didn't know it at the time. Later I discovered they had thought Caesar could be a possible match. I worked with Caesar and Harry, and then Ann went to get Harmony again.

We were *so* pleased to see each other. There was something about Harmony's fine features and white-blonde coat that spoke to me. She was smaller than the other dogs. On first impression, she might be taken for a dizzy blonde. Instinctively I knew there was more to her than that. In comparison, the other dogs were less of a psychological riddle, at least they were not so interesting to me: I wanted to know what made Harmony tick because I had a feeling I already knew.

Harmony and I did the lift sequence which I can only describe as a work of artful choreography – it's as clever as anything you'll see on stage. First, you have to get as close to the doors as possible to block them when they open. Remember, you and the dog are getting in at the same time; also, the dog is on a lead and if he or she gets into the lift but you don't then there's going to be a big problem. Harmony needed lots of encouragement: it was relatively new to her and she had the beguiling combination of being a hapless newcomer supposedly *in charge*, rather like the shop assistant who tells you it's her first day and you have to guide her through the process of taking your payment.

Vicky took us through the lift sequence. Someone came and tried chatting to us (not helpful when I was trying hard to focus), but Harmony and I got through it, not perfectly but safely. I just took to this little soul. We went from the lift sequence back into the main arena, opening and closing doors on the way, by which time I felt more in control, which in turn meant that I didn't have to be reminded not to raise my voice or repeat her name as many times – I could communicate my needs in a way that I felt happy with.

Dogs respond to fun and rewards. *Fun?* I remember questioning this at the very first session with the dogs. How could I get a dog to work for me and have fun? It seemed an impossible task, yet the harder we worked together, the more fun we had.

Now I knew I had a preference, the other dogs just faded into the background. So, how do you know when you've found the right dog? How do you describe that feeling? It's a bit like finding a partner (with a different rewards system, obviously!). There's the first sighting, the crush, followed by curiosity. Then comes the initial spell of shyness quickly followed by all the barriers going down and a sense of uncanny familiarity: *Don't I know you from somewhere? Haven't we met before? Can we see each other again … and again and again?*

After this session with Harmony, I was taken to the animal welfare room where I was tutored in grooming the dogs. An animal welfare nurse called Nicky showed me how to check Elmo's paws and ears.

'*You* are responsible for the wellbeing of your animal,' she told me.

It was at once liberating and empowering to be thrown into the role of carer without any fuss. Indeed, the trainers were remarkably sanguine about our abilities. Their attitude was, '*Of course* you can do it!' That belief translated into our own self-belief. Who would have thought, a couple of weeks earlier, I could care for a dog?

We had lunch while the trainers met for a conference. Joining us was a couple called John and Stephanie accompanied by Stephanie's lovely Canine Partner, Frodo. After 12 years Frodo was to retire into John's care and Stephanie was looking for a new Canine Partner (later I learnt she had been partnered with Elmo and he is nicknamed 'Frodo's apprentice' by John and Steph). They regaled us with lots of stories and in common with Claire, reassured us that it was perfectly possible – and great fun – to live with an assistance dog. Apparently in the early Canine Partner days you didn't learn which dog you had been partnered with until you turned up for the training session.

The day was drawing to a close and now I could scarcely breathe: was there a dog suitable for me? Would it be Harmony, as I secretly longed? It would have been entirely wrong to presume a decision had been made but I couldn't help but feel nervous: I knew we must be nearing a decision even if it was a 'No' because we would have to leave at 4pm to drive to the airport and catch the plane.

Then Ann called us over. She sat down with Mum and me, then announced: 'We think that Harmony is the dog for you.'

'*Harmony?*'

I burst into floods of tears. Afterwards, I hugged all the trainers – I didn't know how to say thank you. They all smiled and looked knowingly: of course they'd seen it all before. Every month, they make these inspired life-changing decisions. It's their job and yet they gain so much pleasure from giving people a new lease of life; they are so kind and sensitive. I felt as if I was joining an exclusive club, where all are welcome.

'What specific things do you need her to do?' Ann wanted to know.

'Can you make sure she's been to Chichester Cathedral because that's where I need to go,' I said, completely off the top of my head. 'I don't want her to start howling when the choristers sing!'

Ann admitted this wasn't the most typical request but she would do her best to give Harmony an appreciation of church choral music. Then Harmony came out and sat on my lap for a cuddle. She loved having her ears rubbed and her tummy tickled; I kissed the fingerprint spot on her head that I'd already come to know and love while Mum took photos. It was the hardest thing in the world, having to go home without her.

Once again, I was too tired to sleep on the plane: over-exhausted but also over-excited, like a little kid at Christmas. Mum and I discussed how to manage things with Melissa and decided that the week before I attended the training course, which we hoped would be in April 2009, we should tell her all she needed to know. There was no point in letting her know too early – the timescale would only confuse her and she wouldn't be able to understand why Harmony wasn't living with us now, today.

At Canine Partners I'd explained to Ann that we would need to write what's called a 'social story' for Melissa. This is a story that explains what will happen, a representation of change using pictures and words. Ann sent me up some photos of Harmony. When the time came to tell Melissa, Ali (my very good friend in Wales) did a lovely social story. It was full of simple sentences and pictures of Harmony to help her understand. Later on, Melissa wrote her own story about Harmony, which we stuck to the kitchen door:

> *Mum is getting a helper dog. I must not give her things to eat. I can help Mummy groom her.*

It was next to Melissa's timetable for each week, which enables her to see what she's doing in big, black letters (very important to her). We stuck pictures of Harmony next to her story so that she could see her and talk about her. Melissa, as you can imagine, was over the moon about having a dog come and live with us. The issue wasn't that Melissa wouldn't like the dog, but that she would like her *too much*. Harmony was coming to live with us as a working dog and she would be a surrogate family pet, not *the* family pet.

'You mustn't feed Harmony, OK, Melissa?' I'd repeat this instruction over and over. Food had to be managed by me, as my way of giving rewards in turn for work. There would be no sneaky Marmite crusts or Jaffa cakes.

'That's weird,' was Peter and Clara's reaction when I told them that they wouldn't be allowed to cuddle Harmony but they were too busy to pay much attention. By then, Peter was studying for his Highers and Clara was adjusting to life at St Mary's as a future instrumentalist pupil.

The weeks raced by. Clara and Peter were excited at the thought of having a dog but the idea was still very abstract for them. It was very real for me, though. Every night, in bed, I'd look at the photos of Harmony and sense myself relaxing: soon enough she would be here with us.

It was another Everest moment.

13

The Pound that Changes Lives

The next three months were marked by feverish anticipation.

Is Harmony really coming to live with us, Mum? Will she really be able to help?

Even her name sounded like a promise. Given my faith and the amount of praying by others that had gone on, I felt blessed to have found her. I had Harmony photos as my phone screensaver; she had become a beacon of hope and her arrival felt like a huge adventure. The sense of mounting excitement buoyed us all up – if you'd visited our family back then, you'd have quickly picked up on the mood. Every time I felt blue or if Melissa was screaming and I felt overwhelmed, I would just shut my eyes and imagine Harmony's big, brown ones gazing at me.

I've always encouraged the family to use humour to deal with my MS – I don't like platitudes or fake cheeriness. When I fall over, my kids laugh. Or if I'm really nagging them, they'll poke me with a finger because they *know* I can fall over! They don't give me any slack because that's how I've brought them up. Sometimes I'll give them a knock and say, 'Sorry, spasm.'

I can be an embarrassment to my family, I'm not going to pretend otherwise: *all* kids feel awkward about their parents. Once on our way out of church, I tripped over the flagstones.

'My, that communion wine must be strong!' observed the resident tramp.

I told the family that I wanted a T-shirt saying 'I'M NOT DRUNK, I'VE GOT MS!' on the front and 'I'VE GOT MS AND I *AM* DRUNK!' on the back.

In future, whenever I had a sense of humour failure I'd have Harmony to pick up the pieces.

In February 2009 I received a pack inviting me to the residential training course. I would have to leave the family for two weeks, starting on 11 April. It would be the longest I'd ever been apart from them and I felt selfish to go away for so long. I had no idea how the kids would feel about being deserted by Mum, even though it wasn't on holiday – in fact, as I would soon find out, it was more like bootcamp for dogs. Once again, I had a long list of commands to learn:

'Up switch!'	*'Open door!'*
'Wait!'/'Behind!'	*'Put it on!'*
'Drop it!'	*'Heel!'*
'My lap!'	*'Get it!'*
'Easy!'	*'Elevator!'*
'Paw!'	*'Fix it!'*

Finding Harmony

'Go to!'   *'Put it in!'*
'Take it to!'   *'Side!'*
'Go in!'   *'Give!'*

After speaking to other partners I learnt that a lot of the dogs respond to the command 'Kiss!' It was just too sweet.

The week before the residential course we went out and bought Harmony a dog bed. I recycled a whole load of the children's soft toys (including Bunny, who is now the sole survivor) and found the old cot duvet in the attic, which we used to line the bed. I was glad to be able to put it to such good use. We were told not to buy too much apart from the bed: Canine Partners would give us everything we needed straightaway and we could purchase anything else later on. Andrew spent a whole weekend building the toilet area in the garden – it was the most elegant dog loo you've ever seen! He put down bark and half-fenced it with spare decking planks. From the kitchen, I'd find myself staring out at it, wondering if it was really true that a dog can be trained to go on command, thus avoiding the need to pick up poo, which obviously I can't do.

Melissa thought it was very funny that Harmony would have her own toilet. She soon lost interest in it, though, when her favourite person in the world arrived in the form of Ali, our friend from Swansea, who came up while I was on the training course. Andrew, who was by now working in Glasgow, had organised time off work to join me for the second week. In conjunction with my

French au pair Aurélie, they had all bases covered and so I didn't need to leave lists. Ali and Aurélie knew Melissa's schedule: I was sure they would be fine.

We gave Melissa her social storybook and informed the school (they had a copy too). By this time I was so frazzled that I felt as if I needed one too: *What's going to happen when I get my dog?* The departure date arrived and it was time to say goodbye. I found it really, really hard and felt very vulnerable about doing the journey myself. *Stop it, Sally*, I kept telling myself. *You can do it. Get on with it!*

I had to dig deep to find the adventurous soul that I knew was buried deep beneath the rubble. It's the disability that makes things scary: if you've been parked somewhere by airport staff and the flight is delayed but no one tells you, then you think you've missed the flight and there's no way you can go and check.

The flight to Gatwick was fine and for once, the staff at Edinburgh managed to supply and use the ambulift (a sort of cargo truck which lifted me up to the airplane).

When we first used it, Peter's response was, 'We always knew you were an old bag, Mum!'

I loved him for that.

On arrival at Gatwick, however, things proved more difficult than anticipated.

'Sorry Madam, your wheelchair is too heavy for us to lift off the plane and we haven't brought a manual, so can you walk from the ambulift, across the tarmac to the waiting minibus and up the steps into it?'

'Er … no I can't.'

'Well, just try! I've got you.'

And so I did my best. Once my knees met the tarmac the crew realised how wrong they were. Even then, it was only when someone accompanying another passenger intervened that they accepted that I needed help. I found myself wondering: *Why do they think I use an electric wheelchair if I could manage to do all these things, to make their lives more difficult or just for a laugh?*

When we got to the luggage collection they deserted me altogether: my wheelchair was beside the conveyor belt, my suitcase going round and round all by itself. Somehow I got the suitcase off, got back in my chair and switched it on and off.

Off we go … Oh no, what's happened?

It transpired the baggage handlers had disconnected the wheels from 'drive' to 'manual'. To repeat the process required someone to bend over to reach the lever underneath the chair to switch over. Once again, someone accompanying another disabled passenger came over and I had to make a phone call to Andrew to ask how to do it. (*Damn, can't I even do this by myself?*) When I finally got to the Costa Coffee to find the pre-booked taxi driver, I was ready for that large latte with an extra shot.

Eventually a lovely lady arrived to meet me. There followed a long drive through the Sussex countryside during which I became increasingly nervous. The sense of new beginnings was everywhere: in the fields full of lambs, the flash of yellow daffodils and the knowledge that I was to see Harmony again. At the same time, I worried she wouldn't recognise me. Would we resume where we'd left off? Was our relationship just as I'd remembered it?

'Hello, Sally.'

I was met by Wendy, the partnership manager at the Canine Partners centre, and shown my room. I'd brought a new tracksuit plus some other clothes and staved off the homesickness by unpacking. I could hear voices as others arrived; it was a Bank Holiday Monday and the training course started on the Tuesday. That evening, I met the other two partners Caroline and Wendy, so there were three of us in total.

Caroline, a fantastic girl who had been very badly injured in a road traffic accident, was there with her tremendous parents, Hazel and Trevor. We cried a lot but we laughed a good deal too for Caroline had a great sense of humour. Both Wendy and Caroline had been through the process before and so I was the newbie. Caroline's first Canine Partner had died and she was now too unwell to manage one by herself so she was to have Giles as a companion dog.

Companion dogs do all the things that Canine Partners do except to go into cafés and shops. Also, the family can take part in exercising whereas in my partnering, I have to do everything with Harmony. Effectively they are special dogs who can cope with extreme disabilities yet perform all the tasks around the home. Dogs tend to become companion dogs if they have a problem with the partnership tasks. For example, Caroline's new dog (Giles) was scared of shops. He was incredible in other ways, though. Caroline took a long time to get words out (although when she did, they were always worth waiting for; either words of wisdom or hilariously funny) but Giles would wait patiently, completely focused on her until she got the instruction out. He was a huge, gentle Golden Retriever.

Wendy, the third participant, was trained in disability benefits so she was a great source of useful information and advice. She was training with her second dog, Yannick. Her first dog (Indie) had had to retire. Usually when a Canine Partner retires, there is an adult in the house so the dog can retire into their care and ownership. It's a system I liked; I couldn't imagine giving Harmony to someone else. Wendy, however, is a single mother and so Indie retired to one of her friends. It soon became apparent that this was a huge loss for Wendy; she also had to manage her replacement dog. Yannick had come from Battersea Dogs & Cats Home (sometimes they will give Canine Partners a call if they think they have an extra-special puppy that might be suitable for the programme). Yannick was a mix of goodness knows what: we were all convinced he had Beagle in him; retriever, too. His ears stuck out and were way out of proportion with the rest of his long body, perched on small legs.

Wendy called him her 'mix-it' dog. She had been told that Yannick wasn't very affectionate but over the fortnight I witnessed how her patience and love transformed him into a dog who loved cuddles from 'Mum'. The training was the same for all of us although I found being the 'newbie' quite intimidating. We met our care assistant,

Yvette, who was always there with us; I only had to utter 'I need …' and already she was producing whatever I needed. Then there was Shirley, the housekeeper: she's the pivot in the residential training course. She doesn't train dogs but she makes sure we're comfortable and feeds us the most amazing food.

That first evening together was spent chatting, unpacking and trying not to feel anxious. After tea, I had to get myself into the middle of a field at the back to get a signal on my mobile phone and see how the family were getting on – I was missing them all. I said hi to Ali, who put Melissa on.

'Is Harmony at dog school?' she asked.

'Yes. How was your day?'

'I love you, Mum.'

'I love you too.'

Afterwards, I went to bed early, exhausted but excited about the following day. The next morning after breakfast, having spent most of the night tossing and turning, I called home again. I was talking to Clara when I saw streams of cars arrive: these were the foster parents (teams of volunteers who care for dogs in advance training over weekends and holidays). They were bringing the dogs back to 'boarding school' after the long weekend. At this point, I saw a familiar face peeking out of the back window of one of the cars.

Was that her?

Moments later she bounded out of the vehicle and I gave her a huge cuddle. How could I have missed her kissing spot and those kohl-rimmed eyes? I don't think we were supposed to have spotted each other, but we did and it was great; I was so relieved that we were both deliriously happy to meet again.

The first day was spent learning about dog psychology: their body language, how to recognise and deal with their fears – canine truths, in other words. We were in the charity's new teaching room. It was big enough for the three of us in our chairs in addition to Yvette and Trevor and Hazel, however add in two or three trainers and the place began to feel like a squeeze.

We learned all sorts of theories that I couldn't wait to try out: we discussed why dogs won't work and why they will, how to make exercise interesting and use body language as a tool for interaction. It was a revelation to discover that I could actually work out what Harmony was feeling by studying her tail and ear positions; also what her fur was doing. At each stage, the trainers tested us: had we listened, had we grasped the fundamental concepts? Each time I reflected back on my previous pets and realised how totally ignorant I'd been of the dog's needs and reasons for behaviour. There are different signs that dogs give off – i.e. calming signals to diffuse a situation, such as very slow blinking or yawning and even, *I'm going to distract you from what you have asked me to do because I don't want to do it* behaviour. The trainers answered our millions of questions and Wendy or Caroline would also chip in with their experience.

At some point during the afternoon bags of dog food were delivered to our rooms. We were given feed bowls that are cleverly elevated on plastic towers, a foot or so off the ground, to make it easier for us to fill them (you don't have to pick them up). We were also provided with a 'vet' bed, which the dogs were used to. Actually, we were given two: one for the training room and the other to be used at night in our room. 'Vet' beds are good as they are machine washable, light and warm: they allow air to circulate. We were also given bags full of the dogs' favourite toys, their coats, harnesses, leads and other bits and pieces.

It was like Christmas all over again.

Harmony had her favourite ball on a rope given to her by one of the puppy parents that Christmas and a soft toy in the shape of a mole. There was also a squeaky toy which we were instructed not to use: apparently it was a method of getting the dog's attention, not a toy. Harmony had two coats, tennis balls, treats, a harness and lead too.

Late that afternoon, at around 4.30pm, Becca and the other trainers brought the dogs out to meet us. They were handed over to us and from then on, they were our responsibility. It was chaos! Twelve paws, twelve wheels and lots of emotion: order was quickly restored when Becca waved us goodbye.

'See you tomorrow!'

Now we were in charge.

'Never leave them and never go out of the centre,' Becca called out after us.

Do you remember the moment when you're leaving hospital with your tiny newborn baby and you realise, *Oh my God, I'm a mum – now what?*

Well, it was one of those moments.

Back in my room, I closed the door. *Hmm*, I thought, looking at Harmony who wasn't sure either (she was used to living in the kennels in the centre). *What's this?* As she looked at me, her ears pricked up.

'Yes, it's you and me now,' I told her.

I negotiated giving Harmony her first meal: I had persuaded Ann to explain and supervise exactly what I was doing. It's really important that working dogs are kept at a good, healthy weight and those of you who own Labradors will know how hard this can be. They like to eat and can easily run to fat. Following this, Ann left. *Hmm, what to do next?* We were looking at each other, each as uncertain as the other.

'And now I think we need a cuddle,' I said, getting down on the floor. 'Do you think we'll be OK?'

Although I might be considered mad to say that Harmony speaks, she certainly communicates (and very clearly, too). Tail wagging, she tucked her head into my chest and then gave me a big lick as if to say: *We'll be fine, Sally! We'll have loads of fun as long as you cuddle and feed me.*

'Agreed!' I hugged her. 'We're going to be fine. Anyway, we have two weeks to get used to this.'

She reversed back and sat on my lap so I could scratch her back. I buried my face in her fur. Harmony loves having her back scratched and sitting on my lap is a favourite position but we were just going on instinct then. As I was getting up to stand, I leant on my wheelchair and the side broke off. In fact, it snapped off with all the controls.

HELP!

I pressed the emergency button. Moments later Yvette appeared and picked me up off the floor. I didn't know what do to – all I knew was that I really needed my chair. Luckily, Gemma (another of the trainers who hadn't yet gone home) brought through a wheelchair with a left-hand control so I now had a strange wheelchair *and* a dog to get used to. Let me correct that: *my* dog. To say I felt scared and overwhelmed would be an understatement.

Dinnertime was chaos as we tried to get our dogs to settle down in the dining room. We were exhausted. Afterwards I went back to my room with Harmony and let her lie down as I groomed her. Then I needed to get back outside into the middle of the field to ring home and speak to the family. I couldn't stop talking: I was on such a high, pumped full of emotion, adrenalin and the excitement of having my new companion, my own darling dog. She was with me, sniffing occasionally and then coming up to me. Melissa kept asking if Harmony would talk to her.

Another first! I ran the bath and got in. At some stage, not long into soaking in the suds, feeling my aches and pains ease and the craziness of the day recede, I realised that I had left my towel out of reach.

Could I, dare I?

'Harmony, get it! Bring it here!' I said, pointing to the towel.

And she didn't hesitate: she got up from the floor, walked over to the towel rail, dragged a towel off it and handed it to me. Success, I was in control of my life! I felt as if we had both been exceptionally clever.

That night I knew she might be a bit unsettled but I got into bed and said to her, 'Go to sleep!' She was very good and did as she was told. In the middle of the night I woke up and coughed; she jumped up, too. We fell asleep in a tangle of arms and legs, which was exactly how we woke up. What joy it was to wake up, no longer alone with the misery of my aches and pains.

That first week of the residential training course we didn't leave the site. It was beautiful weather and the days filled with lessons about dogs and raucous mealtimes just flew by. Talk about chimpanzees' tea parties, it was exhausting! The residential training course is extremely hard work: we were disabled, there for a reason and if one of us burst into tears, saying, 'I can't do another mealtime!' then Shirley was there with comforting cups of tea. She obviously cared about her partners, canine and human.

Remember, a meal wasn't just a meal: we were all trying to eat and working with our dogs at the same time. It's a bit like taking a toddler to a café and trying to eat your sandwich while dealing with his tantrums as the waitress scowls at you. During the fortnight we gradually improved but initially the dogs got in a tangle; like all kids they wanted to push boundaries, leaving us flustered – *and* hungry. Usually a trainer was there to keep an eye on us so that we could sometimes switch off and eat, as well as control our dogs.

Harmony would be endlessly standing up. I'd get her to settle down and reward her but then two seconds later, up she got. 'Settle down!' I would say and reward her, but two seconds later …

'Sally, try not to reward her for getting up,' one of the trainers gently reminded me.

Good advice.

'Just ignore her. She will soon settle down,' was another line familiar from child rearing.

Ignore the bad behaviour. Praise the good.

But learning to do everything properly wasn't so easy. I took Harmony out on exercise while the trainers made sure we were safe – they were always there for support and to make sure that we were doing it right.

'Don't hold the lead – you adjust it but then leave it alone,' said Gemma.

I kept repeating Harmony's name but not giving her an instruction, which they soon picked up on. It was a wonderful thing to feel myself gradually growing in confidence, though. Like proud mums, we were all obsessed with how many times our dogs had pooed and peed. We spent ages saying or rather singing, 'Better go now!' over and over while holding the dogs on loose leads so they could use the toilet area. Of course, after 10 minutes all we wanted to say was, 'For God's sake, *GO!*' The trainers wanted us to see patterns: dogs can do things regularly.

I'd brought waterproofs but didn't need them. In the evenings we shared wine over meals. I texted Andrew, saying: 'bring alcohol'! That same week Caroline's father

Trevor took my broken wheelchair away in the back of his car (he had arranged for someone to weld the arm back on). He really rescued me, which was incredibly generous.

Quite often I'd take Harmony to one of the smaller enclosures at the bottom of the meadow. It was big, but fully enclosed so I felt safe. Exhilarated, I'd let her off the lead and watch her chase dandelion clocks and bark at the shadows. I spent ages grooming her, talking to her, getting to know her. Her favourite thing was to run with us weaving in and out of each other, followed closely by chasing her ball and playing tug.

Grooming she found very boring, and in fact still does. She has an incredibly thick coat that sheds constantly so it's a real struggle to try and control the hair. Once I threatened Wendy that I would send her a cushion filled with Harmony's hair! I start with Harmony standing and gently rub the Zoom Groom rubber brush over her coat to loosen any stray hairs (unlike a comb, this doesn't need to be in the direction of the hair) and then a comb or the Defurminator, a new invention that gets so much hair out, although Harmony doesn't seem to like it much. It's incredible how I never get to the end! I groom for an hour and the loose hair is still coming. During grooming, I also check her pads, teeth, eyes and ears.

Anyway, William's Garden is a wonderful spot at the charity's headquarters that was planted by a volunteer. It's filled with sweet-smelling broom, pansies and daisies; the lawn is beautiful and there is a picnic bench (the dogs stay on their leads there). Like a salve to an exhausted mind, its beauty was our sanctuary. In the evenings we took glasses of wine out there and began our days with tea and sympathy; it was where we opened up about our lives. The garden also offered space for quiet reflection in between exercising and training the dogs. I'd close my eyes and think of my family, hoping Melissa could cope with the change and worrying about them all.

Yes, I was badly homesick!

The middle weekend of the training course was liberating. Shirley and Yvette were there, but no trainers. We couldn't leave the site but what we did was up to us. They stressed that we should rest, which is exactly what we did. We respected each other's need to exercise our dogs by ourselves, slept, read and relaxed.

On the Saturday, Andrew arrived late from Edinburgh. I'd been excited all day – I had missed him so much and wanted to share what was happening, for him to see it all for himself. It was so wonderful to see him again; his soft eyes twinkled and even though he contained his excitement, I could still hear it in his voice. I had reminded him of the 'hands-off' rule the previous day: friends and family have to be trained to sit on their hands. They mustn't pet the dogs nor can they give commands. This is so that the bond between dogs and owners becomes strong. If someone else was more fun or gave rewards, it would confuse the dogs and interfere with that bond.

Harmony was delighted to meet Andrew and had an entirely different take on the hands-off approach, however. *Don't you mean hands-on?* She bowled past me and leapt into his arms, checked him all over and gave him a kiss. Once I had gained a semblance of control and she settled down, Andrew and I were able to talk. He was flying out from Gatwick on the Sunday evening for a meeting in Holland. Before that, he would meet with the others and restock the depleted wine reserves, though.

At the beginning of that week we were taught how to use clicker training. It's a simple method of telling a dog that they are right, if you ask them to do something. They will offer different forms of behaviour until you click so they know that they are on the right track. There followed a hilarious session in which we trained the trainers as if they were dogs. It was comical but also very useful to realise how and when to give clues to your dog.

From the safety of the Canine Partners' site, we then took the big step of taking our dogs out into the big wide world. From Wednesday onwards we began going to shopping centres and cafés. Now we were on our own: the trainers were there but only to intervene in a crisis. This time we had to resolve everything and feel in control in order that the dogs felt safe. Ann was always with me – she had trained Harmony and knew her well. She was my safety net, should I fall (which I didn't).

On the Wednesday the trainers decided Wendy and I should go into the countryside to exercise off-site. I was in the bigger wheelchair. Wendy drove her van while Ann drove Harmony and me. We got out into a big field and I spotted some woods over on the far side.

'Let's head over there,' I suggested.

'I don't think the chair can go down there,' said Ann. 'I'll ask Gemma.'

'Come on, let's just have a look,' I insisted, as I wheeled over to the path. 'Oh, it's not much of a slope!'

'I don't know … Too late, she's gone!' I heard Ann say behind me.

Grinning from ear to ear, I began to have as much fun as Harmony, who had up to that point been rolling in fox poo and getting muddier and muddier. Together, we careered down muddy tracks.

Let's go this way. Can we go that way?

Back at the centre Ann showed me how to shampoo Harmony to get rid of the smell of fox dung (top tip: put a small amount of white wine vinegar in the rinsing water). This was a skill that I would need to perfect, as I found out later. No matter how much she hates the wash, Harmony still forgets the consequences and rolls over and over. Some folks never learn!

During that week we went to a café for lunch and visited Waitrose for shopping. For the first time, we met the general public (by which I mean *curious* public). By now, we had an entourage as Andrew was there, hanging back, never intruding but always there for me. We managed to collect goods from the supermarket shelves and do the checkout sequence. All was going according to plan until I failed to notice that Harmony had spotted a child with a biscuit in a pushchair. Luckily one of the trainers intervened and stopped her from disgracing us all.

Ann stayed calm: 'Just remember to shorten her lead after her task so *you* stay in control!'

Another challenge was lifts so we visited the local hospital, which had big lifts with wide doors. I could not get this sequence right and Harmony looked as baffled as me. *Where are we going? Up or down?* By this time I knew her well enough to recognise the signs that she wasn't happy. She wasn't drooling, not exactly, but she had moist lips and her ears went back very slightly. I became flustered and then finally, we got it right. Becca was there too that day and she devised a way of making it simpler for us: if the lift is big enough, we go in together rather than follow the laborious method of keeping the door open with the chair, getting the dog in, turning round, then reversing and sitting at the back before going in. Coming out, it's best to block the door, get the dog to go through and then leave the lift, especially with smaller lifts to keep the dogs safe. This was all mixed in with remembering to offer our dogs water, allow them sniffing time and all the while being aware of them and their safety.

Lifts completed, we went back to the centre where I enjoyed some much-needed hugs from Andrew and a glass of wine. We were approaching the end of the week.

'What do you want to work on for the last few days?' asked Becca.

'Off-site exercise,' I said.

Now I can't believe how silly I was. Harmony was, and is, as good as gold. And yet at the time, I was terrified of losing her. It reminded me of the lost-baby dreams I had after the birth of each of my children; those dreams in which you get home, unpack the groceries, set the table and then realise you've forgotten something. *Oh no, the baby!* I was scared of Harmony running away, but I was also experiencing the fear of loss associated with having something big and new, something life-changing.

I took away lots of happy memories from the residential training programme and one in particular stands out: Wendy and I are in the countryside with Claire, Andrew and Ann. There's a duck pond and some scrubby bushes. The dogs jump into the pond and have a wonderful swim together, splashing about. I start to laugh at their antics and I'm thinking how good it feels to laugh properly, in such a full, happy way. The dogs scramble out and shake themselves dry. We're all laughing and everyone is soaking wet.

On the Thursday night we had a celebration. It was so warm that we sat outside in the courtyard. As usual, Shirley had done us proud with a magnificent buffet supper. All the trainers and carers were there and we were given certificates to prove we'd passed the course. The trainers came to say goodbye to the dogs and we gave them presents. During the week I had wondered why Harmony sometimes seemed slow to respond: she seemed to think before she acted but I was still annoyed when Ann and Claire commented that I had been very patient with their 'blonde bimbo' and how she was always slow to act. She was my baby, after all!

In fact, her puppy parents also told me she was often the last to do something in training classes: she would watch the others and then it would slowly dawn on her that everyone was looking at her. *Oh, you mean ME, too?* Harmony has a lovely relaxed approach to life unless there's a rabbit or a squirrel to chase. She still has her days when I'll issue a command to sit and she'll respond by fidgeting and looking at the ground. It's as if she's thinking: *Sit, I know that one! Hang on, wait a minute … Hmmm, don't help me, I can do this. Ah, of course, SIT!*

Wendy had come early to talk to us about managing our dogs' welfare. We had been given all the necessary documentation and the vets' books. There was also a report system: I would be expected to send in a monthly report, which included her weight, any attendance at the vet's, any problems that needed to be resolved and fund-raising activities undertaken. I handed over my £1 forming part of the legal arrangement that effectively made me her guardian (Canine Partners retains ownership – Clara always says it's the pound that changes lives). Now I was officially Harmony's proud guardian. I was also given a green disc for her collar that said she was chipped; it has the centre's phone number in case she gets lost. Up until then she had been wearing a red disc, which showed she was a dog in training.

The next morning, a little bleary-eyed and emotional, we had a final mop-up session where we talked about what had been good and bad about the course; also our futures.

I was genuinely sad to say goodbye to Caroline, Trevor, Hazel and Wendy. Together, we'd been through a lot. Andrew and I put Harmony in the car and managed to work out the safety harness (she still makes it hard to get the straps and buckles round her). It's the sort of apparatus that once you know how easy it is then it's fine, but until then it's a nightmare. Like so much to do with having a Canine Partner, it's easy when you know how.

As we headed off into the complete unknown, Harmony settled down comfortably in her vet bed on the back seat.

14

Mayhem and Miracles

We turned left into our road and were met by five sets of eyes at the front window. The welcoming committee waved us up the drive. We'd rung an hour before arriving as we turned off the motorway to say, 'We're nearly home!' I felt just as nervous and excited about introducing Harmony to everyone as they did about meeting her.

'Hi,' I said, climbing out of the car as Melissa, Clara, Peter, Ali and our au pair, Aurélie, rushed out in a mad scrum. I opened the car door, Harmony jumped out and walked into the house as if to say, we're home – there wasn't a moment's hesitation. We put her vet bed into her bed at the bottom of our own bed so that she could smell it and feel comfortable. All the kids brought out their presents (more soft toys) and lined them up in her bed. Like the Pied Piper, Harmony walked around the house followed by a tangle of legs and excitable voices. Melissa pointed out where the loo was, why she has planet wallpaper in her bedroom ('What makes the stars twinkle, Mummy?' is one of her bedtime questions) and how delicious mayonnaise is with chips. She kept asking if Harmony had liked school and pointing out *we* were her family, this was *her* home.

Everyone wanted to cuddle Harmony, which isn't strictly allowed but if you've got three kids and a gorgeous dog, it's a tough call to make.

'Everyone's allowed a cuddle to say hello but let's not turn it into a huge event,' I said.

As I watched Melissa kiss and stroke Harmony, I realised this was everything I'd dreamed of: Harmony had taken on her new home and family without any fuss. Credit has to go to the puppy parents who raised her for the first year of her life with cuddles and proper training. Harmony was fantastic, my superstar!

That night as I tucked Melissa in bed, Harmony curled up beside her. I held my breath: this was not part of Melissa's bedtime routine. Usually if we break the pattern, we run the risk of hours of crying and unsettled behaviour until she finally goes off to sleep. Everything has to be right: no crack of light from the curtains that must be exactly and evenly closed, only one cuddly toy on the bed. The bed covers have to be perfectly folded and the Hannah Montana blanket on top, the right way round, even if it's a hot night.

'Can you read me *The Enormous Turnip*?' asked Melissa, as if having Harmony on her bed for a cuddle was a regular evening occurrence.

Melissa loves being read to and reading itself but her understanding of what's real and what is pretend is limited, which makes choosing books tricky. Her favourite books are the *Smudge* series about animals that live and play together. She knows they're not real because animals don't wear clothes and talk – except maybe somewhere in storyland they do.

'Once upon a time there was a very poor man who planted a seed ...' I began reading.

Harmony snuggled up closer to Melissa. Delighted, she giggled.

'Can Harmony sleep here?' she asked.

'No,' I said. 'Harmony has her own bed but she can stay here until you've fallen asleep.'

It was my first insight into Harmony's wondrously calming effect on Melissa. She accepted this fact with a smile and so began our encounter with the oversize turnip before moving onto *Katie Morag and The Big Boy Cousins*, another favourite book that reminds her of Nannie and Grandad Island's house (my Mum and Dad) in the Isle of Harris.

The next morning, Harmony woke me for her usual cuddle and Andrew made a cup of tea. Harmony trotted into the kitchen and made straight for the bin.

'Yes, that's the bin, Harmony,' I said.

There's nothing like the smell of yesterday's sausages and old teabags to entice a dog to a bin. 'Bin engineering: how does this bin work and how can I get into it?' turned out to be one of Harmony's special subjects. Within days of her arrival, we had to buy a new pedal bin rather than our usual swing version, yet she soon mastered the use of the pedal to flip open the lid, enabling her to dive in headfirst.

'OK,' said Andrew. 'We'll just have to disconnect the pedal.'

'That's a bit extreme,' I said. 'How about moving the bin into the utility room and shutting the door?'

In the end, we did both: the pedal was disconnected and the bin put behind a closed door in the room adjoining the kitchen. Now it was just a matter of remembering to keep the door shut. A week later, I was in the bedroom when I heard creaks and scuffles followed by guilty chomping.

'*Harmony!*'

Rushing through to the utility room where someone had left the door open, I found Harmony eating the remains of Clara's Cornflakes, which had been tipped from the bin onto the floor.

'I saw her do it,' said Aurélie, who was in the process of sweeping up.

Yes, this time my clever Harmony had stood up on her backfeet, grabbed the bin between her front paws and tipped the contents (spaghetti, cereal, more teabags) into her mouth – and onto the floor.

'*Go to bed!*'

Perhaps I should have got wise to Harmony's bin fetish at the Canine Partners' residential training course, where she'd put her head in the bathroom bin and then appeared wearing the lid like a necklace. Looking somewhat sheepish, she had wagged her tail enthusiastically. *Look at me, silly or kind of cool?* It was a 'you-should-have-been-there' moment: I didn't have my camera but it made me laugh. Luckily the bin wasn't stuck on her head for too long.

Another purchase made over the weekend was a new 'Henry' vacuum cleaner. No way could the old one cope with the mass of hair that sticks to the carpets every day. My beautiful purple and burgundy carpets have both taken on a golden hue – so much for my request to Wendy all those months ago! I laughed. It reminded me of the training course when I wore my brand new black track-suit for Nicola's grooming lesson. Everyone thought I looked hysterical in my hairy outfit and yes, I felt a bit foolish.

Saturday morning and I knew that I must take Harmony for a walk. It sounds silly, but I'd become fearful of the idea. I could feel the dread building up: I was scared of losing my dog.

'Just do it!' said Andrew, with typical straight-forwardness.

As usual he was right. It was a gorgeous morning, the big two were still asleep, Melissa settled and I needed to get over my fear. Besides, we are lucky enough to have a park and woodland just a 10-minute walk from the house.

'Will you come, too?' I asked.

'Of course,' Andrew smiled.

Now I could relax: I went in my shop mobility scooter. First, I took Harmony to the toilet area with the instruc-tion, 'Better go now!' She peed but was clearly deter-mined that was it. We turned right out of our street and left into the main road that takes you into the city centre. Harmony walked alongside: she knew exactly what to do, following my commands. She seemed completely relaxed, unconcerned by traffic, the boy who whizzed by on his bicycle or the convoy of prams and screaming babies. We crossed at the lights and turned into the park.

As soon as Harmony got wind of the smells of all the other dogs, her tail began to wag. Once we'd got past the trees and were in the park, I let her off the lead. She and I always use the controlled release we had been taught: I get her to sit and then wait. I take off her coat and harness, wait a bit longer and then release her. And I felt so proud that we managed it: I didn't need to worry either – every time I stopped my scooter or called her, she came straight back. She wanted my approval and of course I had the tube of cream cheese, just in case.

Each time she ran off in the direction of a fresh scent and a new adventure, she'd return, ears pricked, to let me know what she'd been doing. *You'll never guess what I've just seen? A squirrel, but I can't work out where it went. Hey, come and look at this! I've found the oak tree where all the other dogs have sprayed.* I'd only been in the park for 10 minutes yet already I felt the emotional lift that Canine Partners talk about: to see Harmony sprint through the trees, her hind-legs bouncing in the air and screech to a halt like a crazy cartoon dog made me laugh out loud.

Why had I never done this before? All those months and years of being trapped indoors, too depressed and overwhelmed by my frozen legs to leave the house for a simple walk in the park. It had never even occurred to me to go for a walk in the woods. Now look at me!

That night, Harmony may have been dreaming of squirrels as she slept in her bed beside Andrew and me. Every so often she'd make a whinnying sound and shudder. I'd amuse myself with thoughts of her chasing squirrels in her sleep.

Sunday. I knew green fields were the best place to do some obedience work with Harmony. This involves recall training, which is when she waits for me to return to her. We also practise wheelchair positions or loose lead walking and walking to heel with no lead in these sessions. I'd discovered that I really enjoyed this type of exercising; I felt she and I were learning all the time and the obedience work continued to establish the boundaries of our relationship. I also wanted to prove to everyone that my 'blonde bimbo' could do it. Her 'emergency down!' – if she runs into trouble this is used to establish immediate control; for example, if a bike or car suddenly appear or I need to take control – is still slow but we have managed to reduce the time lag considerably. Having said that, when it really matters she never lets me down and has always dropped immediately, as instructed. Say, for example, the game has got too boisterous or someone is trying to control their unruly dog then I always get a thrill when Harmony comes immediately and sits by my side while we wait for the other owner to gain control (butter wouldn't melt!). I do remind admirers that I was given Harmony as a fully trained dog, though – I really can't take all the credit.

* * *

More importantly, now that I'd rediscovered the big outdoors, there was no holding back. We drove out to a private estate now in the council's ownership called Cammo. These beautiful grounds include patches of wilderness, derelict buildings and a canal that begs to be swum in by dogs. Woods, trees, open fields ... it has it all. Once again, I couldn't stop smiling.

The year we moved back up to Edinburgh, Andrew and I both bought Barbour jackets, mine ankle-length. Barbours last forever and they're impermeable to Scottish rain on *dreich* (rainy, miserable) days. It wasn't raining but the Barbour was the perfect foil to the cool country air as we tootled about. Andrew, as always, patiently walked at my speed: he never put me in the position of having to catch up, even in my walking days. The smell of wild garlic and the sight of bluebells were a reminder of my past – my years as a walker, a climber. Tears pricked my eyes as I realised I hadn't seen them in more years than I cared to remember and I might never have done so, if not for Harmony. Andrew too was quietly content; suddenly things had improved.

Oh dear, where was she?

I called out her name: 'Harmony!' and she came instantly. After that episode, I learned to relax, confident in the knowledge that she would come back. Indeed I marvelled (along with other dog-walkers) that no matter what she was doing, if my scooter stopped then she would suddenly appear to check up on me. Recently, on the same walk I called and this time there really was no response. I called again, trying not to worry, and she reappeared. She then stopped to sniff a bush and gave me an impatient look that seemed to say: *Yes, I'm coming in a minute!*

'No reward for you, Miss,' I told her. 'Just because you're a teenager doesn't mean you can behave like one!'

I would have to teach her. After returning in a minute, she soon got the idea when she was rewarded with carrot rather than cream cheese (which is for an immediate return). These days, she comes at once every time but doesn't know if she will get a reward – it's all part of the game.

Puppies and young dogs, especially if they are Labradors, eat everything. They chew shoes, devour cuddly toys and consume whatever they can shove their faces into. I'll never forget Sandie eating my sixth birthday cake, the Christmas cake and various other cakes in between.

A week after Harmony arrived home, Melissa became 10: she hit the double digits and we were to celebrate by taking her and some friends from Funky Monkeys (her special needs group) plus a bunch of others from her class on a narrow boat. It was a special boat that had been adapted for wheelchair-users by the charity, Seagull Trust. They run narrow-boat trips and have a specially converted boat for hire, enabling disabled users to access our canals.

Melissa had already specified her cake of choice: choco-late, with Postman Pat on it. I was so tired after the two weeks on the residential training course that when Ali offered to make the cake, I thanked her and went off to take a nap while the kids were at school.

The cake went in. Thirty minutes later, Ali got it out of the oven and left it to cool while she went out into the garden to make some phone calls. Half an hour later, there was no cake: just one very happy dog, with crumbs on her chin.

Ali was in tears.

'*Harmony!*' I said, eyeing my new companion ruefully.

But I wasn't going to shout: our training had followed the cardinal rule of never shouting, always praising. After all, she was a Labrador and Labradors eat cake; it had been too tempting for her to resist.

'You have let me down,' I told her in a low, stern voice.

We didn't tell Melissa for it would have brought an abrupt end to a blossoming friendship. Food is as important to her as it is to Harmony. Instead I put on an apron, reheated the oven and baked another cake. This time it was left to cool on a high shelf, well above Harmony's reach. It was a reality check: a reminder that I was living with a dog, not a saint. There would be many more such reminders to come.

Melissa couldn't wait to introduce Harmony to her friends at school. Again, this posed something of a dilemma: I didn't want the children at the school gates to feel they couldn't approach Harmony or that they should be afraid of her, but at the same time they had to know she couldn't be touched or fed. Before I left for the residential training course, I had informed the school that I would be bringing my assistance dog to the school gates but she wasn't a pet and I needed the kids to know this. I followed this up with a letter to the headmistress, asking for her help.

Ultimately, the school was magnificent as were the kids on that first afternoon when I took Harmony there (it's less than a mile from home).

'That's the dog we can't touch,' they said, pointing at her.

Meanwhile, the mothers at the school gate studiously ignored me because they had been told to ignore the dog. Then I waved and they realised that I wasn't entirely off-limits and it was possible to interact with me while respecting Harmony's role as my Canine Partner.

At this stage, Melissa was a pupil at a regular primary school with a special needs facility. The school was brilliant at injecting fun into her extra groups: Funky Monkeys. Two of her best friends at Funky Monkeys were Stuart and Caitlin, who have Down's syndrome. It took about two minutes for me to realise I'd have to lift the touch embargo rather than attempt to explain to the two of them why they couldn't say hello to Harmony Instead I let them greet and pat her, which made them feel special: they were allowed to touch Harmony! It brought smiles to a lot of faces.

We'd had big family discussions about how I would maintain Harmony as mine: she had to remain my assistance dog rather than the family pet.

'Hey, *I'm* the one with the rewards in my pockets!' I said.

Indeed, you can't avoid the smell: I'm the one with poo bags and soggy Kibble (dog-treat mix) in all my pockets, which makes for horrible brown soapsuds if they get into the washing machine. Equally disgusting is the stench of rotten sausage in the car.

After a day of country air and keeping up with Harmony the weekend after Melissa's birthday, I was so exhausted. I flopped into my comfy chair in the living room – a big recliner with a footrest – to go through the schedule for next week. Who would pick Clara up from school on the Wednesday after her rehearsal? Melissa had to have a new swimsuit (she had lessons on the Wednesday) and Peter needed some cash for the millions of things that the school wanted money for.

Melissa started to scream. She stood in the doorway leading to the living room and let out a scream from the top of her lungs. I have no idea why. It could have been the sight of a spider lowering itself from an invisible thread or a spot of blood on the au pair's finger. It might have been distant sirens as ambulances hurtled to an emergency on the other side of the city.

Without prompting, Harmony got up from where she was sitting beside me, walked over to Melissa and very gently leant against her. She sank to the floor and Harmony planted herself in her lap. With this, she wrapped her arms around Harmony, buried her face in fur and stopped screaming.

It was a miracle ... another miracle!

Andrew, Clara and Peter came running out of their rooms and looked on in amazement. We were absolutely stunned: Harmony was obviously the right dog for us all.

Finding Harmony

Months later, when I told Canine Partners about Harmony's healing effect on Melissa, they said that she had shown similar intuition as a tiny puppy. While not yet a year old and living with her puppy parents, the very young son of friends had come for a sleepover. The little boy had recently lost his mother. Sensing his sadness, Harmony didn't leave his side all weekend.

It was then that I also found out that Harmony had been intended as a guide dog for the blind. Occasionally, there are exchanges like this between charities with a dog unsuited for one role who might do better elsewhere, or the charity has too many puppies at that time (as in this case) and so they offer them to other assistance dog charities for purchase. When Harmony was spayed, the vet nicked one of her veins and it wasn't certain if she would live through the night. Somehow my miracle dog survived. Also, she was very nearly partnered with a lovely girl called Sarah, who was eventually partnered with Harry (one of the dogs that I had worked with on my assessment days and her second Canine Partner). Sarah's first Canine Partner was an assistant called Hazel. She and I have remained in contact: we both agree that H's are the best and have christened ourselves the 'Nearly Mums'. Fate could so easily have intervened on many occasions to prevent Harmony from being mine, but we got there in the end.

Harmony quickly became Melissa's new best friend: if she was worried or having a bad day, she'd ask for her. When it was time for her booster jabs (Melissa hates needles), Harmony came too.

She was one of us now.

15

An Expanding World

'I'm redundant.'

'Don't be silly, Clara. Of course you're not.'

Clara and I were settling down to an evening at home; Melissa was finally in bed. Exhausted, I had dropped into my reclining chair and Clara was next to me on the settee. We had our laptops open for some Facebook time while watching TV (I think it was *Desperate Housewives*, an addiction Clara had introduced me to). In the past I would usually drop the remote, or the phone or my mobile. Clara would get up, retrieve it for me and settle back down only for me to ask her to take off my slippers and socks. Up she would get and so on for at least the first half-hour of any evening together.

I hated it: I hated knowing that Clara would have to get up and down for me at least three or four times before we could relax.

Now that I had Harmony, I could settle down with my trusty treat bag and she would do all the work for me; I could resume control of the remote and the running of the house, of my life. By the time we were slouched in front of the TV, Harmony was just as happy to rest as me. These days, after a couple of requests to fetch socks and mobiles, she will raise an eyebrow: *You're joking, right? I mean, look at me. I've only just got settled – I'm comfy.* She releases a big sigh and gets off my lap (yup, she still considers herself a lap dog) before taking off my socks. Then she gets back on my lap. More sighs. I love Harmony being on my lap. It only took her a few weeks to work out where to position herself so that she could dampen down my spasms; she has her tongue ready for a comforting lick on my hand whenever it goes into spasm.

Harmony's arrival meant a shift in family dynamics. Previously, I had depended on Andrew and the eldest two children to help me dress in the mornings and put down my footplates. If I'm honest, the task of helping had fallen less to 18-year-old Peter and more to Andrew and Clara, otherwise the au pair. Now I had Harmony and no one needed to bend at my feet to put down the footplates for me or lift my legs up onto them; no one else had to put my socks on and or take them off either. In case you're wondering, the reason why I have socks endlessly taken on and off is because my feet are incredibly uncomfortable. They feel as if they've been stung by bees: it's a hot-scratchy-freezing-cold-numb feeling and it drives me mad.

Clara, more than the others, had felt responsible for me in a way I hadn't chosen for her or anticipated. It's one of the well-documented side effects of living with a sick parent: in effect, you become the parent of your own parent. At the same time it was part of our very loving relationship. Clara is a hugely compassionate girl who feels a deep sense of injustice (inherited from her parents) at the plight of children who suffer and people's prejudices.

One summer we went to a performance of the Scottish Opera's *Cosi Fan Tutte* at the Edinburgh Festival Theatre and I went into spasm. This isn't pleasant for me or anyone watching: my heel looks as if it's trying to reach the back of my head, my right arm whacks anything within reach (usually Andrew, which the kids find hilarious for obvious reasons) and I grunt. I'd forgotten to take my evening medication: 10 tablets designed to reduce spasm and pain – I have to take them by eight o'clock or all is lost.

'It's all right, folks,' announced Clara, extremely loudly. 'She's forgotten to take her tablets!' It made me laugh and the folk around us less uncomfortable.

Afterwards, Clara pushed me up the hill, her high-heels clacking as she chatted away about the performance: why the musical arrangement wasn't as dramatic as it should have been, who was to be in the jazz recital at school and why algebra is so cool (apparently, it's great fun to rationalise formulae!). Clara loves school.

On the other hand, Peter's idea of helping Mum is to start sprinting with the wheelchair, while yelling, 'I'm running away with Mum,' as I scream and hold on for dear life.

The last time we visited Lauriston Castle, just outside Edinburgh, he decided we needed the exercise together. Not only was I stuck in my wheelchair, now I was in a boggy field and howling with laughter. Peter walked away, hands in the air, as if to deny all knowledge of how I'd managed to get myself into such a ludicrous situation. Peter is our clown, as is Harmony.

Anyway, what I needed to convey to our daughter that evening in front of the TV was that Harmony's arrival would make our relationship simpler: closer to the type of mother-daughter connection that didn't involve having to get your mum dressed or grabbing a glass out of her hand when her arm went into spasm. I didn't want Clara to have to second-guess me all the time. I was keen for her to be able to be a teenager; to sleep in late at weekends and worry about *her* life, not mine. And yes, life for Clara has become easier but it doesn't stop her worrying. The big change is that she and I now have fun: Harmony has restored my sense of fun. I embarrass my daughter and we have our normal tiffs, but that's life. After all, she's 15 and I'm her mum.

Harmony has paved the way for all this and more, although she hasn't quite got the hang of making tea, mixing a gin and tonic or catching a mug before I hit the deck. Once I'm prostrate, she comes and checks me over. It's as if she's grumbling: *Oh please, pull yourself together! Do you really need to lie on the floor again? Haven't you done enough of all that?* I can feel myself being lectured for not being sensible. For me, the joy was the realisation that Harmony loves helping me: she wags her tail, rushes to claim rewards and seems to think it's all a great big game. When I tell people that my dog gets the washing out of the machine and gives it to me to hang up, they always laugh and joke, 'I could do with one of those!'

An Expanding World

Mind you, one load of washing is OK and two is tolerated but after a heavy washing day, we get to load three and Harmony looks at me as if to say: *You're taking the Mick here – I mean, this is ridiculous! No one needs this amount of clean laundry.* To avoid the need for industrial arbitration (i.e. Harmony making a formal complaint to Canine Partners), I up the reward level to cheese: she'll do anything for cheese. Again, this is working on the high-and-low reward systems. Tiny slivers of cheese or liver cake or sausage are high rewards that the dogs will work extra-hard for; carrot and broccoli are low rewards, with which Harmony seems equally delighted. If I'm going somewhere new or asking her to take on a job that's harder that usual, I'll up the reward to encourage motivation. In some ways, it's not dissimilar to bribing my son with chocolate to get my newspaper from the newsagent!

Two weeks after Harmony arrived, I decided to take her to Sainsbury's. The supermarket is a 20-minute walk from my house and part of a shopping complex. In general, Andrew does the weekly shop at weekends or on extreme occasions online, but I needed a few things for myself. More importantly, I wanted to test the boundaries of my independence and feel as capable as any other person to move freely outside of the house; I was also keen for Harmony to keep up her range of skills (I knew she didn't like shopping very much). As my health deteriorates, I will need those skills more and more.

I dressed Harmony in her purple jacket with 'PLEASE DON'T DISTRACT ME – I'M WORKING' clearly written on it in big white letters. Then I got into the wheelchair, did my customary keys-purse-lead-rewards-bag check and we left the house. Mandie, my aftercare worker from Canine Partners, had come all the way from Ayrshire to be with me for this momentous occasion.

If you have a growing family or have had babies then you'll know what I'm talking about when I say that the organisation and determination needed to leave a house is monumental. To hear the click of the lock as the door shuts behind you is an Everest moment. As usual, I took Harmony to her toilet area with the instruction: 'Better go now!' This is done so that she'll feel comfortable (one of the reasons why the dogs won't work for you is if they need to go to the loo). Usually Harmony looks at me and politely refuses the offer just by standing there. I have since learnt that she has the most enormous bladder but in the early days with the Canine Partner Rules ringing in my head, I'd stand and wait with her for sometimes hours. It was very stressful and not dissimilar to toilet training toddlers: once they've gone, you make a mad dash for the door and head for the shops to optimise the time.

We arrived at Sainsbury's and began trundling up and down the aisles looking for shampoo, gluten-free bread plus bits and bobs. Luckily the aisles are wide enough for a wheelchair and dog.

'Oh, what a lovely dog! What's her name?' asked a lady with a big smile, her hand outstretched and ready to pat Harmony.

'Sorry, do you mind if you don't,' I said. 'She's working.'

'Oh, I'm terribly sorry!' she frowned and backed away.

My beautiful blonde Labrador means I'm no longer invisible. Before I had Harmony, I *was* invisible. In fact, I once embarrassed a gentleman in the local shop who was buying a bottle of water and leant over me in my wheel-chair to pay.

'Oh, I didn't see you there,' he said, as his coat sleeve brushed against my hair.

'My invisibility cloak works very well when I'm in my chair,' I told him.

Now I've gone from being invisible to being ultra-visible and I have to deal with the general public and their inability to connect the message on Harmony's jacket with my dog.

PLEASE DO NOT DISTRACT ME

'Oh, but I can, can't I?' is a fairly common response; 'Oh, but I can't resist,' being another. The two other most common questions are: 'What can she do for you?' and 'Do they get to be an ordinary dog?'

I don't doubt most people have the best intentions but when you're trying to remember all the commands (you need to get your working dog to go past the checkout, stop, take your purse and then pay for the groceries), it's incredibly distracting to have to fend off the over-enthusiastic public at the same time. At Canine Partners we were taught techniques on how to cope; also, how to see trouble coming and avoid it, and if you can't avoid it and can't get the message across, how not to be rude.

After all, we are ambassadors for Canine Partners. On the Facebook page for human and dog partnerships, we share our experiences of dealing with the general public. It's not uncommon for someone to write that they have been refused admission to a café, or to have had their dog (who is in the middle of a task) drop the packet of biscuits in response to being stroked with the result that you have very crumbly biscuits by the time you get to pay.

Another frequent comment is that it takes us twice as long to do anything because people talk to us about our dog. Yes, at last, not the wheelchair but to *me* about *my* assistance dog.

We were taught to give our dogs a false name for the first few months so that no one would call them on seeing them again. Sounds harsh but it's true: people will call out to your dog from the other side of the road just as you are negotiating traffic light sequences, buttons, beeps and cars.

I once had a lady approach me to say, 'I really shouldn't do this – I used to puppy walk for Guide Dogs for the Blind,' and proceed to blithely stroke Harmony. 'Oh, but she is *so* irresistible!'

'*PLEASE*, stop doing that!' I insisted.

A few minutes later, she zoomed in again but this time I was quicker and moved my wheelchair between her and myself so Harmony was out of reach.

'Oh, what's her name, how old is she?'

By now I was intently studying the label of a packet of pasta (sometimes being hard of hearing has its advantages). Bionic eyesight, however, is an essential tool: it's amazing the number of old ladies who carry dog biscuits in their handbags! You see them from miles away rustling their bags and twitching excitedly at the sight of Harmony. One of my tricks is to say to Harmony, quite loudly, 'Don't touch!' which the old ladies think is directed at them and so they back off. Otherwise I avoid eye contact and manoeuvre the wheelchair into a different direction.

Back at Sainsbury's, I managed to find what I needed on shelves that weren't prohibitively high (Harmony had been able to retrieve everything) and we made our way to the checkout. Before I began putting my groceries on the conveyor belt, I asked the girl, 'Are you OK with dogs?'

'Yes,' she said.

She totalled the goods and Harmony jumped up with my purse.

'Oh no, we're not allowed to take customers' purses,' she said, shaking her head.

'But she's an assistance dog,' I persisted. 'It's her job.'

'Sorry,' said the girl. 'It's shop policy.'

Now I was cross. Not wishing to cause a scene with a queue behind us, Mandie and I moved to the Customer Service section.

'Can I speak to the duty manager?' I asked.

The manager duly appeared. I introduced Harmony and explained my situation.

'Canine Partners are new to Scotland,' I said. 'They're like guide dogs. I don't understand your policy about purses.'

'It's just our policy.'

'Well, do you think you could possibly organise a meeting about dogs in purple jackets and point out the difference between dogs in purple jackets and those without?' I continued.

Mandie then asked if we could use an empty checkout at the other end of the shop, far away from everyone else, in order that Harmony and I could practise the checkout sequence.

'No,' came the reply.

My confidence now in tatters, I left my shopping – and Sainsbury's. I might have Harmony but it was still me against the world. Then I went to Marks and Spencer, via a patch of grass for a sniff break, where the girl took my purse from Harmony's mouth and I got my lunch. They could not have been more welcoming; they were kind, helpful and amazed by Harmony. Boots the Chemist was next. They had just redone their store but guess what? There were no low-level counters at the checkouts; they were all too high and narrow for Harmony to jump up.

On the way back we stopped at George's, the newsagent, to pick up my newspaper. Harmony pushed open the door, I pushed it behind her and in we went. By now she knew to ignore the tempting smells of crisps and chocolate and make her way directly to the counter.

'Hi George,' I said, then turning to Harmony. 'Up table!'

Just then the door opened and a big gang of schoolboys came in, laughing and joking. They shoved their way to the front, unaware that Harmony and I were in the process of working together. At this point I should have left the overcrowded shop. Stubborn as I am, I chose not to.

'Up table!' I said again, this time too loudly.

Flustered, Harmony leapt and landed with her four paws on the counter. Her intention had been to stand up on her hind-legs and offer George her jaws, in which to take the paper. There was silence and then George burst out laughing. Realising her mistake, Harmony slid down backwards, ashamed, having retrieved my newspaper.

'Good girl!' I told her, as we made our way out.

It is still one of George's favourite stories. He is incredibly kind and helpful. We've now trained Harmony to go into the shop alone, pick up my newspaper and head out. I still worry for the safety of those Mars Bars and Snickers on the bottom shelves but so far, so good.

When I think back to the six months prior to Harmony's arrival, I often spent entire days alone without speaking to anyone. As anyone who has ever suffered from loneliness knows, it's debilitating. I always tell my doctors: I've suffered from depression and I suffer from MS but I know which is hardest: 'the Black Dog', as Mr Churchill used to describe it, is infinitely worse. However, within a week of having Harmony and taking her to the local woodland, I'd found a community of dog-walkers, who I soon came to call friends. Whatever the weather, I was now spending at least an hour in the park every day during which I shared stories, daily moans and canine truths with a trusty bunch of friends. I had rejoined the working world – I had a daily gossip, just like everyone else. Everyone has their good and bad days but by sharing your woes, no one's left feeling down. Among our group, there have been shoulder fractures, births, deaths, illnesses, exam success and failures.

'Hello, Harmony.'

It was Liz, the owner of a wonderful Flat-coat called Barney. He has a gorgeous shiny coat and brown eyes that sparkle with mischief. I'd met Barney and Liz on the very first Monday when I went to the park to exercise Harmony without Andrew. Barney is beautifully behaved and of course, reminds me of Guy, who I worked with at the Canine Partners' centre. He is taller than Harmony and just as obsessed with squeaky balls; he is, however, much better at remembering where he's left his ball! We have had coffee at Liz's house a couple of times. The chaos of toys scattered around the garden is a reminder of play-dates with toddlers. Other children's toys are so much more fun and interesting than your own: Harmony loves Barney's toy box.

Harmony and Barney hit it off immediately. Off they ran, beating a path through the undergrowth, before racing back to tell us where they'd been.

Hey, we ran all the way to the bench and chased a pigeon!

Then Barney lifted his leg and peed all over the two front wheels of my scooter: now we were as good as family.

Liz and I have worked out various routes across the park: taking different paths and directions to avoid boredom for both the dogs and ourselves. She happily takes paths that can accommodate the wheelchair, as do all the dog-walkers; she tells me about her day and children, and I tell her about mine. When we reach the junction of trees where all the paths intersect, one of us always comments we need a café, right there. It would make the perfect stop for a cappuccino break with a bowl of water for the dogs.

'Oh, look who's here!' I find myself waving.

I soon built up a network of dogs and dog-walkers that I looked forward to seeing. There was Eric and Dorothy, with Mangus and Buddy (two gentle, older Retrievers) and Martin and Lee, with their Spaniels, Dino and Desmo (Dino loves to drop his ball onto my scooter). In fact, all the dogs make a beeline for Eric, who seems incredibly popular. Obviously if you happen to be carrying a particularly tasty, smelly treat then you'll soon find yourself surrounded by dogs, all vying to be 'Best at Sitting' in order to gain a treat. None of the dogs are encouraged to play with sticks, but balls are the norm and it isn't unusual to lose one in the bushes and find another.

'I don't think of you as Sally with MS in a wheelchair,' said Liz, after a couple of months of knowing me. 'I think of you as Sally with Harmony.'

It was a lovely thing to say – especially as she had had to push my scooter with its dodgy battery a couple of times to get me up the hill. Whenever it was serviced, the mechanic would sigh and say, 'Sally, it's called a shop mobility scooter for a reason!'

Most days after dropping Melissa off at school, we make it into the woods by 9am. Harmony's other best friend is a Red Setter called Sara, who is owned by Muir and Norma. Muir is always nagging me that I should take more care; that I'm too reckless and wild on my scooter (I'm like a teenager on a skateboard!). Then there's Anne and her two large Spaniels, Will and Ben, and an incredibly patient lady Eleanor who rescued one of her dogs from a breeder and had to teach her everything, from enjoying grass to socialising with other dogs. As the weeks and months passed, you could see the dog transform and gradually relax until it was able to run and meet the other dogs – she still keeps very close to her owner, though. Joining them is a young Red Setter called Brea. As a young dog, she loves to play and bounce. It makes me laugh when I see Harmony pretend to be too grown up for this whippersnapper. There are no obvious alpha males or a leader in the pack, however: the dogs all greet each other and off they tear.

It seems I'm not the only one to think of Harmony as a shy schoolgirl.

'All Harmony needs is a boater set at a jaunty angle and she could be a St Trinian's schoolgirl with those freckles and that cheeky smile!' declared Liz.

Harmony is the youngest of the pack and the newest recruit. If the pack gets too big or her beloved Barney plays with someone else, then she will hang back and watch. Mind you, she doesn't hang back if there's a stick in sight! She loves chewing sticks but this isn't good for the dogs as splinters can get stuck into their soft palate or throat. Sticks are something of an obsession with Harmony, though. One day, she was chewing on what must have been a particularly delicious stick and she simply would not let go. In the end I threw it into the middle of a prickly bush and Liz and I moved on with the other dogs. Harmony followed and as far as I was concerned, the stick was forgotten. Oh no, think again! On the return journey, we passed the other side of the bush and off she went into the thick of it to retrieve *that* stick. This meant Liz had to come to the rescue and disentangle her from a particularly thorny branch, which managed to get caught up in her collar. Eventually, Harmony reappeared, triumphant, clutching the stick in her jaws.

In the early days, the chief difference between me and the other dog-walkers was that they came armed with plastic bags for picking up poo and I didn't. Now it's not quite true: over time, Harmony began to work out when I was going to exercise her and would refuse to use her toilet area. She tilts her head coquettishly, which is as good as shaking it, and does a little shrug.

No way! I'm not going now with you hovering over me. Besides, why should I go now when there are all those big bushes waiting for me in the park?

Fortunately, I can now reach over my chair far enough to pick up the poo if necessary and if I can, so too can others. It really annoys me when I see excrement lying on pavements or in the grass – it gives us dog-walkers a bad name. Having said Harmony won't go, she will if I haven't exercised her yet and we need to go shopping. Clever girl!

The only other difference at the park is that the other dogs are free to tear off and behave like dogs. Harmony, in contrast, always has one eye on me; it's second nature to her. Every few minutes, she'll come back to check up on me. In return, she still needs my protection and reassurance when the pack becomes too unwieldy and she feels overwhelmed. *Mum, look after me*, she pleads with her big brown eyes.

At the end of the summer, Liz and I were just finishing our walk and having our customary moan about the lack of a park café when we heard Anne call for help. We couldn't quite hear what was wrong but as we turned the corner we spotted her. One of her dogs (Will) had collapsed. He was elderly and Anne had told us that she was worried about him – in fact, he had an appointment with the vet that very afternoon.

We hoisted him onto my scooter. Anne walked alongside, one hand cupped to keep his head up. Liz had Barney, Harmony and Anne's other dog Ben on their leads. Together, we made a slow procession to the gate, where her husband was waiting with the car. It turned out to be Will's last trip to the park for he died that day at the vet's. The next day, the dog-walking community were ready with cuddles and solace.

The following week, my scooter developed a puncture halfway through the woods. The wheelchair lurched to the right but not hard enough to throw me out. Luckily, Martin and his wife Lee were there; Martin supported me to the gate while Lee and Cath, another dog-walker, pushed my scooter. I rang Peter and was met by my son and his girlfriend at the park's gate with the manual wheelchair to get me home – thanks, team!

16

Double Trouble

One of the things that I hate about being disabled is that it's impossible to be spontaneous. You can't say, let's go to London this weekend or let's see a movie tonight and even well-planned travel is not risk-free. Often I'll ring up a restaurant or hotel to see if it's possible for me to go there.

'Do you have disability access?'

'Oh yes, we're disability-friendly,' they insist.

But then I get there only to discover there's a flight of steps to reach the front door and the downstairs bedroom has a floor-level camp bed. Add to the mix Melissa's needs and you'll understand why a trip away makes for spontaneous combustion rather than fun. The fact is, we're not like other families so we can't just get on and do things in the way they can: I'm in a wheelchair and Melissa is like a toddler; she needs constant supervision. She has to know where each of us is, all the time, and she can't abide change. If Andrew wants to put up shelves, we have to send her to Granny Edinburgh's. The sound of a drill and the banging upsets her; she just doesn't have the analytical skills to understand why she's distressed.

Monday to Friday is dominated by routine: school, swimming, tea, bed. Saturday is pancakes with Dad; Sunday is always church. One of Melissa's favourite places is the Yard Adventure Centre, which has the biggest sand-pit in the world (I'm not joking!). Designed for children with disabilities of every kind and their carers, it has its own stream and a bed that's a swing, with room for 10 kids to lie inside with pillows. There's a sensory room, arts and crafts; also a kitchen for the carers to make them-selves a cup of tea – it's about allowing children their inde-pendence and enabling them to organise themselves and make decisions about what they want to do. Kids can wander there. When I bring Melissa back from the Yard, she's a different child: she will draw and play in the garden by herself as opposed to asking me to do it with her.

Melissa adores the zoo (particularly the monkey house) and she loves public transport: a bus ride to the zoo, followed by tea in a café is the dream ticket. Each year, her grandparents buy her an annual zoo-pass for her birthday. I was worried that Melissa's world was becom-ing increasingly small and mentioned this to her granny. She now takes her granddaughter on buses and to the shopping centre, where they go up escalators and visit the cinema. Melissa can't follow a story but she loves the music. *The Princess and the Frog* was a bit hit: it's set in 1920s New Orleans and has fantastic jazz that makes her eyes gleam. It can be a bit awkward because she loves to get up and dance! We have learnt to go to the cinema during off-peak hours and also, to time our arrival so the trailers and adverts are finished. Otherwise Melissa asks,

Double Trouble

'Is it finished?' when the ads have come to an end but the feature film itself hasn't actually started.

In October 2009, we decided to go away for the weekend in the Highlands. We had prepared Melissa, packed everything she needed in order to feel safe and happy, to occupy and prepare her for the change. Her pillows and torch? Tick. Monkey? Tick. Her books, DVD player and DVDs? More ticks. We also packed for Harmony and already we knew her extensive list off by heart: food, whistle, treat bag, bed, towel, two coats (in case one gets dirty), leads, harness, food bowl, toys and Bunny (by now a sort of security blanket). We were to stay in a ground-floor flat with stunning views over a lochside with sand and shale beaches.

Autumn in Scotland is stunning: thanks to that year's Indian summer, the leaves had changed colour late in the season and the trees were a collage of russet reds, bitter oranges and sunburst yellows. The loch's waters reflected the sky; cotton-wool clouds skudded across the brilliant blue as a gentle breeze ruffled the waves. Overhead soared birds of prey. Rabbits ran for cover and in the distance we spied deer, startled by our footsteps.

The beach isn't the easiest place to be in a wheelchair, nor in fact was the flat. But what the flat lacked in disability access, it made up for with stunning views. I knew that at some stage over the weekend, I would be left sitting on the beach in my wheelchair, watching the others in the distance. Which was exactly what happened: sometimes you must bow to the majority while partaking as much as you can. Melissa wanted to fish from a little wooden jetty but I was keen to take Harmony and the family for a walk along a forest track. This time, however, I drew the short straw: jetty, it was.

So there I was, stuck in my wheelchair on the beach, feeling increasingly isolated and frustrated. Not only had I lost my family, but I'd also lost my dog. Everyone else had walked down to the end of the jetty, they were having fun and that made me happy; what worried me was that Harmony had disappeared and it was her first experience of a sandy beach, with all its briny smells. She loves swimming and it was hardly surprising she'd wandered off. I shouted for Andrew.

'I can't see Harmony!'

'Don't worry,' he told me. 'I can see her.'

'What's she doing?'

'She's digging in the sand.' He paused. 'It looks like she's eating something ...'

'Oh dear,' I muttered.

He went to get her. Harmony played with the family for a while, then disappeared again. When it was time for lunch, we made our way back to the flat. We packed up and left for home with lots of happy memories.

That night Harmony fell ill: she was groaning and quite clearly in pain. She had eaten rubbish in the park before and been sick. I'd always stuck to the Canine Partners' rule: starve the dog for 24 hours. If the complaint continues, take her to the vet. Harmony kept stretching, arching her back and making the choking sound that accompanies retching; nothing came out. By this stage there was just bile. She wouldn't lie down or sit; she was just standing and swaying.

I spent much of the night up with her, rubbing her tummy and feeling helpless, not knowing what to do.

Tuesday morning, I took her to the vet. I love our local vet: The Oak Tree Vet Centre. We know all the vets at the practice – they have treated three past rabbits and the current duo, Duchess and Snuffles. They even managed not to snigger when the white rabbit turned out to be female (I had booked both rabbits in for neutering!). They've saved rats (Peter's teenage pets) and even sorted out the ferret when our short-term fostering became long term and I couldn't stand the stench, so had him neutered. Oh yes, and once the ferret fell and hurt his paw: cue another trip to the vet's.

This was worse, much worse than anything I'd experienced before: Harmony was now an extension of me. Would she be OK? It was almost as if I was taking a child to casualty.

'Her stomach is full of something,' said the vet after a brief examination. 'I can feel something that feels like pebbles. We'll need to take an X-ray, which means giving her a general anaesthetic.'

Terrified, I signed the consent form and asked if I could be with her.

'No, go home and we'll call you when she is ready for you,' he told me.

I went home and rang Canine Partners. Wendy wasn't available but a kindly voice that picked up the phone triggered a wave of sobs from me.

'It's Harmony! I've had to leave her at the vet's for a general anaesthetic and X-ray. She's eaten sand and won't stop being sick, and I am so scared and feel so guilty!'

She listened while I sobbed. Then Andy, the chief executive, called me back. I kept apologising but he continued to reassure me that dogs do these things (she's a dog not an angel, remember?) and told me to keep in touch and let them know when I had more news. My parents were visiting and they waited with me. It was a very long day.

Finally, there was a call.

'Harmony is awake now if you'd like to come and collect her.'

I raced round there. Before Harmony was brought out to me, however, I was taken through to the vet for the news.

'The X-ray is showing a considerable quantity of sand. It has moved from her stomach to her bowel,' he told me and showed me the X-ray.

I could see what looked like an enormous stuffed sausage, in a stuffed bowel.

'She's digested approximately three kilos of sand and stone,' he continued.

I could even see some stone shapes in the X-rays; it looked painful.

'So, that's what she was eating,' I said.

Later on, we decided that the sand must have been covered in fish guts, which accounted for its particularly delicious flavour (sand alone isn't that tasty!).

The vet sent us home with laxatives and instructions to feed Harmony regular small amounts of oats but by the next day, to my consternation, she hadn't recovered: in fact, she seemed to be getting worse. Now she couldn't stand up. She was severely dehydrated and refusing to eat or drink so we took her back to the vet's. Something was really wrong if Harmony was refusing to eat. It transpired that there was no point in doing a stomach wash as the contents were all in her bowel. An enema carries its own risks. The other problem was, as the vet put it: 'What do you get if you mix sand with water?' Answer: concrete. Her bowel was severely impacted.

They kept her in for the day and fed her intravenous fluids (she was sedated again) and planned to give her vast amounts of laxatives. I was really worried about leaving her and tried to explain to the vet nurses that she wouldn't perform on concrete and needed to be given specific instructions – 'Better go now!' – and did they have a toileting area that she would be able to use?

At the end of another very long day, the vet's called me to say, 'You can come now.' This time, Harmony did look brighter but there had still been no bowel movement. They had managed to get her to eat a little by tempting her with moist food rubbed onto her gums and sent me home with the rest of that tin and two more. 'Keep up the laxatives, mix in lots of oats with the meat and keep an eye on her,' were the instructions. I was to bring her back in the morning for another appointment.

Then I took her home.

Not only did I feel grief-stricken but I felt guilty at having neglected Harmony: I had allowed her to eat sand. I called Canine Partners to apologise again and report on her status. They were very supportive and understanding (which only made me feel worse).

To maintain her high-roughage diet, I fed her little bits of the expensive tinned meat with oats, just lots and lots of oats. There was still no action when we revisited the vet. 'Don't worry,' they reassured me. 'It will happen eventually.'

Day Five. Hallelujah! Things moved – and kept moving – for days. Being mostly sand, her stools were too crumbly to pick up, but still it was progress. All in all, Harmony was out of commission for 10 days and I missed her dreadfully. It brought into sharp relief how much I needed her: she was physically present, but emotionally absent. She had no energy and was too sore and uncomfortable to jump up onto the bed so my rest times weren't the same. I kept lying beside her, trying to hug her.

On day 10, she jumped up on the bed for a cuddle with a sock in her mouth. I burst into tears.

'I've missed you,' I kept saying. 'How I've missed you!'

They say dogs can't tell the time but when, at 5.27pm, she started to pester me for her grub I knew she was better – and capable of reading the hands on the clock.

That Christmas was very special. As usual, we opened our stockings on the bed and I immediately realised my mistake: Harmony didn't have one. A few seconds later, I handed over a hastily wrapped biscuit.

Although Clara was no longer in the choir, she and Andrew had taken part in a radio recording, in which she sang a small solo. Andrew, Clara and Peter sang in our friend Dean's church, a wonderful, small Episcopal church with the most loving and welcoming congregation. It was Church of the Good Shepherd's Nine Lessons and Carols. On Christmas Day, Andrew and Clara (wearing a cassock) sang together in the cathedral. Melissa, Harmony and I sat in the congregation. Clara had solos and it was a beautiful experience.

When it came to communion, Melissa scampered up to the altar rail before I could stop her.

'I want Jesus too!' she insisted.

Then she sat down beside her dad and had a big cuddle. Afterwards, I apologised to Dean, the vicar.

'I wish everyone was as keen to take communion,' was all he said.

January 2010 and still no sign of a thaw. Snow is fun for kids and snowboarders, but it's a hazard for old people and wheelchair-users. In fact, the ice was so severe that I couldn't leave the house. I'd no choice but to relax the rules on me being solely responsible for exercising Harmony – I was simply unable to take her out. Instead Andrew, Peter and Clara had to put on boots and scarves to take her over to the park.

Tuesday morning and the sun began to creep out from behind the clouds; the birds that lived in the wood were singing, the animals would be out foraging. It had been three weeks since I'd felt the wind on my cheeks. If it was warm enough for birdsong, it was good enough for me.

'Come on, Harmony,' I said, getting myself into the electric scooter and yanking my coat off the peg. 'Let's go!'

Finding Harmony

I found her coat and put it on; as I transferred myself onto the scooter, I slipped but managed to right myself. Following this, I adjusted Harmony's lead to the right length, did my key-purse-mobile check and left the house. I was apprehensive, but how bad could it be? The pavements had been gritted, the sun was out and at some point you have to leave your anxieties and your house behind. It felt wonderful to be outside, breathing in the cold air. We made our way down the main road and Harmony pressed the light at the crossing.

'Good girl!' I told her and gave her a bit of Kibble as a reward.

We crossed the road and entered the park, following the gritted path that led into the woods (this route allowed me to get into the top woods without using too many slopes). The paths had cleared, there was not a drop of snow in sight and we were enjoying ourselves, which in retrospect was what gave me a false sense of security. To give you a brief sketch of the park, I should tell you there's a slope between the woods that you have to descend in order to reach the grassy park at the bottom. There, I could do some obedience training: Harmony hadn't done any recall work for weeks and I was keen to get things back to normal. I had missed my fresh air and our work together. If we kept going, it would give us a circular walk.

But I'd forgotten about the sheet ice. I got to the top and felt the scooter start to slide; I tried to turn back. Too late! We began to skid, or rather to fly down the hill backwards.

Double Trouble

It was more a case of 'Let's *goooooooooooooooo*!' than 'Let's go!'

Life went into slow motion. *Right, Sally*, I remember thinking. *You've got your thick padded coat and your gloves on. Put up your hood!*

At the last minute, the scooter hit something, spun and I flew out of it.

Luckily, one of the care assistants from Melissa's old school spotted me from an upstairs window. She ran to get her coat on, thinking she could at least help with Melissa if she was there but once she saw that it was just me and had been reassured that Andrew was already on his way, she went home. I had landed in a ditch with the scooter on top of me. I remember my head hitting a rock with a clunk and thinking, *OK, that wasn't too bad*. But then I passed out.

I came to (I'd been unconscious for probably no more than a couple of minutes) with Harmony beside me, howling and barking away. A couple walking their Golden Retriever were standing next to her. Apparently Harmony had been running to and fro between us to alert them to my accident, just like Lassie. I had been calling out too, it seemed. The couple lifted the scooter off, but wisely didn't try to move me.

Andrew appeared.

I'd called him from the ditch to say I'd had an accident although I have absolutely no recollection of this, which was disconcerting. The couple had already called an ambulance and within minutes, paramedics in green appeared and set about examining me. Harmony was very distressed: she kept getting in their way and barking at them. Andrew put on her lead. Then they lifted me up and put me onto my scooter (it was far too dangerous and icy to carry me in a stretcher). They got me to the waiting ambulance by holding me on the scooter while Andrew pressed the lever to make it move.

Harmony went ballistic as I disappeared into the ambulance and the doors shut. Later I found out that Andrew had had to pick her up and literally stuff her into the car. He took her home for reassurance and cuddles although she then lay by the front door until I came home, some hours later.

At the hospital they ran some X-rays. Despite having landed on my right side (my bad side), miraculously I hadn't broken anything. However, I had to have the gash in my head glued and there was bruising under the surface of my skin. One of my frustrations is no matter how hard I fall, I never seem to have a bruise to show for it. Afterwards I was extremely sore and had a cracking headache for days.

Harmony and I were both traumatised by the fall. For months afterwards, I had trouble getting her in the car; she associated it with separation and it triggered fears of all sorts. Over time, and with judicious use of treats, she returned to herself.

I am still terrified of that slope but I refuse to be beaten. We do it as part of our routine walk, both up and down, with my lovely dog-walking friends walking quietly beside me. When we get to the top, Harmony walks backwards in front of me to check I'm OK. Liz and the other dog-walkers are amazed by her intelligence and technique. If I have trouble with the scooter, she stops and comes back again to make sure everything is OK. And if she hasn't seen me for a while, she needs to sniff me – it's her way of checking me over from top to toe to make sure I'm in one piece.

She worries about me – it's her job.

17

Venturing Forth

'Melissa, what's your favourite game?'

'Hide and seek: I hide then you say, "Sit, wait!" while I go and hide; then you say, "Go and find Melissa!" and Harmony comes and finds me.'

Melissa loves playing with Harmony: her level of trust in her means that she also communicates through her. If she is scared or confused about something, she will say, 'Harmony is worried about the sore leg', or 'Harmony doesn't want to go shopping'. We respond to her concerns by talking to Harmony, through her.

'Tell Harmony that the leg is getting better because the Band-Aid fixed it, so she doesn't have to be scared.'

Sometimes we ask Melissa if she really means that Melissa is scared of something, but the risk here is that by talking directly to her about a subject that scares her, she will panic.

We're a tactile family: we love cuddles. Melissa would sit in my lap all day if she could. She also loves putting her face in Harmony's fur – it calms her down. I'll put my arms around the two of them, which often leads to

Venturing Forth

Harmony reaching up on her hind legs and putting her front paws on either side of my shoulders for a cuddle. She started doing this in response to us cuddling each other. When anyone comes home we have a hug, but I didn't realise that Harmony had been watching us.

One day, Andrew came home. Harmony waited for me to have my cuddle and then she jumped up and put her paws on his shoulder ready for her turn. She thinks of herself as a member of our family – it's lovely to watch. Harmony has bonded with me and will choose to be with me, wherever I am, but that doesn't stop her from having cuddles with the rest of the family. She loves her tummy rubs from Peter, hugs with Andrew and back scratches from Clara (she appreciates her strong musician's fingers). Harmony also picks up on our moods, especially mine: if she is worried about something or concerned about me, she will put her head between my knees and just stay there. If she picks up on any feelings of sadness or pain, she will lie beside me with her head on one of my shoulders, licking my hand, long before it starts to spasm or stops working altogether (which can go on for a day). After a big spasm, I can even fall out of my chair. I'm gradually getting weaker and more spasms now occur on a weekly basis. It's as if Harmony understands what's going on – I just don't know how.

As I have mentioned before, Melissa doesn't relish change, which means that she doesn't like going on holiday – in fact, she finds it very stressful. We've recently started to go on city breaks (we've visited former au pairs in Berlin). Melissa goes to stay with Granny and Grandad Edinburgh (Andrew's parents) and Harvey, their Cocker Spaniel (Melissa's other best friend). Harvey is immensely patient with her, Granny devises outings and we leave knowing Melissa is happy.

This year it was Bulgaria and the first time I'd left Harmony. I was so excited about visiting a new country, going abroad, but at the same time I was worried about leaving her behind.

We were to drop her off at kennels near Biggar and they came highly recommended: the owners of Sara, the Red Setter we walk with, use them for all their dogs. I'd looked up their website and I liked the ethos, the small-ness and the fact that the owner uses the profits from the kennels to fund her animal rescue work. Being a coward, I asked Peter to accompany me on the hour's drive. We were delivering Harmony the day before we left. I felt so miserable.

'Don't worry,' said the manager, as she returned from taking Harmony to her kennel. 'She has gone in like an old pro – she'll be fine.'

And so she was.

Once again, Canine Partners proved their brilliance in preparing the dogs for all eventualities and had actually sent them off to kennels for regular kennel breaks. As it turned out, Harmony was perfectly well behaved and not unduly concerned (you hear stories of some dogs chewing the bars of their cages). When we picked her up, Bunny was still intact so we knew there had been no anxious chewing.

Venturing Forth

We had a fantastic weekend in Bulgaria. Peter and Clara specifically asked if we could visit a country about which they knew nothing, somewhere new, and somewhere neither Andrew nor I had been to. I had booked a ground-floor flat and emphasised that I was a wheelchair-user. When we got there, we discovered there were 15 steps to the front door! The ground floor turned out to be the first floor. Steps aside, we had a superb time, discovering the old and the new: beautiful churches and scenery intermingled with communist-era buildings. We were staying in a refurbished flat in one such block and the central heating was communal so we couldn't choose when to have it on or off.

We flew home on the Sunday night. Officially, I wasn't allowed to pick up Harmony for another 12 hours. The kennel rules are very strict: no collecting pets after hours to avoid people turning up day and night, but I was desperate to see Harmony and so I took a chance and rang ahead.

'We'll be passing your door at about nine o'clock tonight. Can I come and get Harmony?'

'Yes, of course you can,' said the kennel owner. 'Usually it would be a problem but not this evening.'

Joy! We arrived, Harmony was brought out to me and we had an emotional reunion – you'd have thought we'd been apart for months, not days. I insisted on sitting on the back seat with my dog and cuddled her all the way home.

* * *

I felt encouraged by Harmony's response to being left in the kennels and in doing so, I'd also recovered my sense of self and my place in the world. Sod the MS, I could go anywhere, do anything and off-the-cuff! MS is progressive. I am marking the deterioration weekly, which means that I'm keen to do as much as I can *now*. Last summer, we went sailing at the Culvert Trust at Kielder. It has a huge forest and the biggest manmade lake in Europe. I sailed by myself for three hours, in a specially adapted sailing boat. The others were water skiing. Oh, the glory of rushing along in the waves, feeling the wind in my hair, the sun on my face and doing it all by myself. (Indeed, my Mum tells me that my most oft-repeated phrase as a toddler was, 'I do it myself!')

But there was a penalty: as soon as my feet touched the ground, I was subjected to all-over body licking from Harmony as she checked me over. It was as if she was grumbling: *How on earth am I supposed to look after you if you go off and do stupid things like sailing by yourself?* As I've become more adventurous, her grumbles have got more vocal – the family find this hilarious. We headed off through the woodlands looking for the Wave Chamber (an architectural installation by the lake).

'You can do a lot of the activities here, but you will never make the Wave Chamber,' warned the man at the desk when we arrived at the Culvert Trust.

The family groaned. Obviously I'd *have* to go to the Wave Chamber now.

We set off. I was in my scooter, which as I've said before is designed for trips to the shops and not off-road adventures in muddy woodland. It took my whole family to move rocks and part trees, pushing and shoving me through bogs; the scooter by this stage was somewhat worse for wear (obviously I need a vehicle designed for more extreme terrain!). I got there in the end and took the photos to prove it. The Wave Chamber was a tiny, hollow cairn with a smooth floor that catches the sun; it ripples and makes the sound of crashing waves. Once inside the chamber with the door shut, you're treated to an amazing sensory experience.

The next thing I knew, Clara and I had booked flights to Amsterdam for the Easter holiday. It was our first trip away, just the two of us; it had been her idea (I'd always wanted to show her Anne Frank's house). Clara had just read Anne Frank's diary and was keen to visit the annexe where the family had hidden. I'd also enjoyed the diary when I was 13 (the same age as Frank, when she began writing it) and found it as poignant and haunting as Clara had. Finally, I managed my dream of visiting her attic home when I was 42 and on a trip with Andrew, with him lifting my leg up the steps. This time, my MS was far worse, though.

'You will have to go in by yourself, sweetheart,' I warned Clara, in advance of our trip.

'Are you sure you'll be OK if I leave you?' she asked, worried.

'I'm sure.'

We arrived at Edinburgh Airport and the girl at the check-in looked at Clara and enquired, 'Has *she* packed her own bags?'

Finding Harmony

Clara turned to me and asked, '*Mum*, did you pack your own bags?'

It was a fantastic 72-hour, whistle-stop tour of Amsterdam's cultural hotspots. We managed to use the goods lift to get me onto the canal barge; we visited the flower market and the Royal Palace, as well as hidden gems such as the best apple pie shop and the oldest distillery in Amsterdam. Clara had the map and planned out all our routes and itineraries. She pushed me over cobblestones, took the hump-backed bridges at a run and even managed to cross a busy intersection (even though I did end up in a pile of builder's sand when she drove my chair into a pavement under renovation, but that's another story!).

We stayed in a wonderful B&B in the Jordaan district, a 10-minute walk from the Prinsengracht Canal and Anne Frank's house. The manager, a lovely lady called Charlotte, explained when I rang that there were two small internal steps and a grab rail that ran down to the ground-floor bedroom. It was exactly as she had described it: brilliant!

I did think, as Clara knelt to help me undress, *I need my dog*, but Canine Partners don't allow us to take the dogs abroad (although each request is considered on a case-by-case basis). The stress on the dogs would be too much. Besides, this was my time with Clara. We laughed and chatted and had a great time.

Andrew took time off work to look after Harmony and Melissa. The trip made me realise that not only is it possible to travel, but how important it still is to visit different places and explore the world. It was such fun seeing a new city, discovering its history and culture and sharing it with Clara.

Then it was back home.

Sometimes Melissa's needs are overwhelming and our four hours' respite a week, recently allocated and managed by the Lothian Autistic Society, is a huge help. Even with this, it's a battle. There are no shortcuts or easy answers yet when I spend time with Melissa, it never fails to amaze me how much of life I see. She forces you to slow down: you can spend hours in the garden with her looking at ladybirds and counting petals on a rose; there's a joy in living life in the slow lane – it's a positive thing. It makes me realise how fortunate I am in so many ways.

'*No*, Harmony – I don't need my sock taken off!'

Oh dear, Harmony is bored. I'm working and she wants to be working (and have a reward). If she can't work, she's just as happy playing tug o' war with me: she has to remember not to shake her head so when she's tugging me up from bed or shutting a door (all a variation on the tugging game), she won't injure me (or her). She's like a professional Gun Dog or Retriever in the way that she has to look after her jaws except no self-respecting Gun Dog would ever play tug.

Recently, a bored Harmony found a new way to get my attention: she walked over to the table and knocked a book off it in order to retrieve it and give it to me, tail wagging, eyes sparkling.

Finding Harmony

Can I have my reward now? I just picked up that book, didn't I?

Busy working in the summer of 2010, I found myself regularly presented with my shoes and her lead.

'OK, Harmony, let's go!'

We were on holiday and had found a lovely walk, leaving Melissa with Ali and her friends in the nearby paddling pool. I joined them after the walk: we watched the kids play and had ice creams. Suddenly Harmony decided enough was enough, so she pulled my sweater out of the scooter basket and gave it to me. Then she pulled her coat out and gave that to me, too. Having completed this task, her brown eyes shining, ears pricked up and head tilted to one side, she seemed to be saying: *Please, can we go home now, or DO something? I just hate sitting around!*

Harmony is quite funny these days in managing me: if she picks up a dropped item or starts to empty the washing machine, she won't release the item from her jaws until she's *sure* there's a reward in my hand – she's no fool! I've learned to be faster with the rewards.

Recently I've written some articles for the press about living with an assistance dog and even been filmed for CBBC (*Animals at Work* will be broadcast in 2011). My kids simply roll their eyes.

'Oh you and your tragic life!'

'It's not tragic at all,' I tell them. 'I've had an amazing life – I've seen Everest, I've travelled through China and I've got a wonderful family and Harmony!'

Now, if Harmony sees a cameraman she will start doing all of the tasks one by one, like a performing dog.

It's hilarious. In May 2010, Canine Partners wanted to do some promotional filming and so we went to spend the day in the Pentland Hills. All of a sudden, I felt a tingling on my right side.

'I'm going into spasm,' I said.

In a flash, Harmony was at my side, licking and cuddling me. Afterwards, I asked if the cameraman had got it on film. But no – he had been far too astounded and moved by Harmony's ability to comfort me to keep the cameras rolling.

A few days later, I was moaning to a Canine Partners' friend on Facebook about my MS and being in a wheelchair when she made the point: 'But you wouldn't have Harmony if you didn't have MS.'

And it's true. Harmony has restored my sense of fun. I have to get up and get out – and I have someone to cuddle when the family are out getting on with their own lives. Harmony dissipates the everyday sadness that comes from being disabled and in pain: my gatekeeper, she keeps the tentacles of depression from descending.

She's also restored my taste for adventure. In June 2010 we flew to Southampton together to do some work for Canine Partners and have a team photo. It was Harmony's first flight. I felt very nervous but I'm always ready for an injection of Heyshott, to talk about Harmony and be among the trainers – it does me the world of good. As usual, Edinburgh managed to mess up the arrangements and the ambulift wasn't ready for us. Instead, the flight attendants decided to board all the passengers first. They then had to manhandle both me and another passenger (who was hemiplegic) onto the plane full of passengers with less space.

'OK, Harmony,' I said. 'We can do this.'

Harmony was terrified, crossing the bridge from the ambulift to the plane. Once in, I had to pull myself along the seats, holding onto the backs, until I got to mine. It was a long shuffle: I felt the eyes of everyone on the plane on me, which is never easy (and something I'll never get used to). Feeling hot and bothered, I got into the seat and tried to get Harmony to settle down but there was no space: Harmony lay at my feet, about a centimetre into the aisle. The next disabled passenger was brought in and the assistants rolled the stretcher chair over Harmony's tail, causing her to yelp.

I wanted to cry. However, it seemed the whole plane was sympathising with poor Harmony. Eventually I got her to, 'Go under!' the seat and moved her out of harm's way. The rest of the flight was uneventful: Harmony was happier about crossing the bridge into the airport now that she had done it once and we walked into the terminal. I was so happy to see Jill from Canine Partners standing there with a big smile.

Off we went to Canine Partners' headquarters. Gosh, it was good to be back at Heyshott! Becca came out to greet us, showed us our room and rustled up some lunch. Harmony wanted to jump up. I was *so* embarrassed (did they think we'd forgotten all the rules?).

'Harmony, *OFF*!'

She was just so pleased to see everyone. Then, as we assembled for the photo-shoot, I could sense Harmony was becoming tense and unsettled; she wouldn't curl up beside me. Instead, she kept standing and nudging my hand. I was absolutely shattered and so off we went for a rest. By now, Harmony was clinging to me, giving the odd little whine and constant licks and cuddles.

One of the trainers – Ann, Harmony's original trainer – offered to take her for her night-time toileting.

'Come on, Harmony!'

But she wouldn't leave my side and suddenly it clicked.

'Harmony, I'm *not* leaving you here,' I said, bending to stroke her. 'We are just visiting! You're coming home with me again.'

I'm sure she thought that returning to Heyshott meant she would be left behind, that our time together was over. I was filled with emotion – it told me everything I needed to know. We were a team and she needed me as much as I need her. That night, full of pizza and wine, I snuggled up next to her for a good night's sleep. (*But don't tell them she stayed on my bed all night, especially don't tell Shirley. It's a secret, OK?*)

The next day we flew home: this time, all the staff at Southampton made it incredibly easy, though. Harmony was relaxed crossing the bridge and we didn't have an audience to distract us. I put her into the seats first so she was properly tucked away and she soon settled down.

'Due to operational reasons we will be delayed by about 20 minutes,' announced the captain.

Great! Eventually we took off. When we arrived back in Edinburgh, I was as usual forced to wait for the ambulift. (An international airport with *one* ambulift? Please get it together! All the disabled people and airline crews I have met agree Edinburgh is the worst for care.)

But then the captain came out and said: 'Hi, I'm your personal chauffeur! I flew you down yesterday and brought you back today. Where shall we go tomorrow?'

I loved it: someone was cracking jokes with me. Mind you, my mood soon changed when he explained that the reason we had been delayed was because a member of staff had a serious allergy to dog hair. Ah well, it was almost a triumph!

Harmony's official passing-out parade and Partnership Day were held in September 2009. In the November, Ann came up to Edinburgh to study her progress and to do the final check. If we passed this test, Harmony would be permitted to wear the full coat and no longer required to have 'IN TRAINING' on her back. I've lost count of the number of people who ask me who it is that I'm training her *for* – this always makes me smile.

The appointed day came and I was so nervous. That morning, I took Harmony out for a quick run in the woods so that she would be calm and rested. When Ann arrived, we chatted over life in general and the difference Harmony had made to me. We displayed our task work, went to the shops and demonstrated road safety and shop tasks. Following this, we went on exercise and I showed off our obedience work – I was so proud of Harmony as she did everything she was supposed to, a really clever little girl!

Venturing Forth

We came home and Ann looked at Harmony's record book and conducted a physical check. She wanted to make sure that I'd been using the flea and worming treatments regularly (not only are these important, but also required by Environmental Health as she has access to public spaces such as restaurants and cafés). Ann explained that if Harmony was over- or underweight, or if I hadn't been caring for her, this was an immediate fail.

We came and sat in the sitting room while Ann scribbled in her file. Have you ever sat quietly while an examiner notes something and you're trying to read the writing upside down? Well, it was just like that! I could feel my heart beating in my throat: I knew Canine Partners can, and will, 'fail' partnerships in their final assessment and continue to work on trouble spots until the eventual pass but I didn't want that to happen: I was eager for our partnership to pass because I felt so confident in it.

'Do you want the good news or the bad news?' Ann eventually asked.

My heart sank.

'The bad news is that you now have to give your old coats back. The good news is you get new ones!'

The family, who had been hanging around all this time and pretending not to listen, erupted into cheers. We all hugged each other – and Harmony, of course. I was so proud of what we had achieved: during the training course the trainers had drummed it into us that it took six months for the dog-human partnership to become established and I'd secretly thought, *yes, whatever*. But now I'd say it's six months plus: it's a gradual process that you don't see happening but when it does, it's absolutely seamless.

Partnership Day: this was held before our final check in November. It's a chance for the trainer to talk about the dog, for puppy parents to see their dog and partner and any sponsors of a dog (it takes £10,000 to get one of these dogs into a partnership) to get to meet the partnership they have sponsored. The partner can also talk about the difference having a dog has made to their lives.

I was so excited! Andrew came with me; other partners stayed there, too. I had a new outfit for the occasion (a purple jacket and skirt – a bad choice as it instantly showed all Harmony's hairs) and was supposed to have a speech ready. The night before, I scribbled a few notes. *Oh heck, whatever was I going to say?* Usually I have no problem with public speaking but this was different, this was Harmony's day.

I looked out at a room filled with hundreds of people.

'The first thing I have to say about Harmony is I asked for a dark-haired dog who didn't moult,' I said, casting a glance at her.

After the laughter faded, I went on to explain what a perfect match we were and how impressed I'd been by the matching process. I told everyone about Harmony, her character and all she has done for me; I also talked to them about Melissa and the transformation in our lives. Then I thanked everyone involved in Harmony's training and care for without them this would not have happened.

I was so very proud of Harmony and our partnership that day. The puppy parents had brought puppy photos with them and told me lots of stories – it felt as if they were filling me in on the bits I'd missed. It turned out that one of Harmony's early puppy parents has an autistic son and another has a trumpet-playing daughter.

During our team photo, I dropped my pen (I pretended I hadn't noticed as I didn't want to get Harmony to pick it up in front of all those people). I was so nervous about things going wrong, despite the fact that at home she would do everything without a moment's hesitation. As I set off, the puppy parents pointed it out.

'Is that your pen, Sally?'

Harmony had to retrieve it, and of course she did so successfully.

Naturally, there were other dogs there, too: all of them were special and had amazing relationships with their partners. I was moved to see and hear about Glen's dog Geri, who is dual-trained. He is a Hearing Dog for the Deaf and a Canine Partner as Glen is both disabled and deaf. Now that's a clever dog! There is also a partnership where the dog is dual-trained as a Guide-dog for the Blind and a Canine Partner – it's amazing what the charity manages to do with its dogs and skilful training techniques.

Nine months after Partnership Day, in June 2010, Canine Partners celebrated their presence in Scotland with a gathering of the five people in Scotland who now have dogs, plus the many supporters. I took Melissa and Clara. We were welcomed into the lovely home of Suzette Rankin in Tullibody, Perthshire. All of the fundraising committee were there, as were those who have been generous with their time and money. Andy Cook was there in his role as chief executive too. I had been asked to say a few words about Harmony.

'No leads, it's the dogs' party too,' said Suzette, when she met us at the door.

What a brilliant idea! Suzette has a huge garden that resembles a country park. It was a glorious place for the dogs, who soon found their way through the trees and down to the Lochen (a mini-loch or lake).

I'd put on a floral skirt and a pretty top. As Clara recently pointed out, my wardrobe has changed since getting Harmony: no longer do I buy exclusively black (mourning) clothes. We were all outside in the garden and I'd asked Clara if she would agree to talk about how much a Canine Partner changes the job of a carer and about her own caring role. She was also providing the background music with her *clàrsach* (harp). It was the first time that she had spoken publicly about Harmony, but Clara is such an assured speaker and she was just superb. I felt so proud and moved, listening to her talk to the garden of about a hundred people, telling them: 'My mum has always been my rock but I had to help her a lot too, now that I am a teenager ...'

'Thanks, Clara,' I said, afterwards, aware that people were pointing and beginning to giggle although I didn't know why. Suddenly, out from behind me tore a pack of dogs, including Harmony: the five partnered dogs and all the supporters' dogs. They had been in the Lochen and were soaking wet! After bowling up the hill, they waited until they were in the middle of us and then shook themselves dry. Cue an outburst of screams and squeals. It was a good moment and a timely reminder: Canine Partner dogs are allowed to be dogs, too.

I hadn't planned to become a public speaker yet through finding Harmony, I'd found my own voice: no longer was I invisible for I had an assistance dog and a story to tell. Around this time, I began to give other talks to help raise awareness of the amazing work that Canine Partners do and to highlight my case. At a lunch for a local garage that sponsors a Golden Retriever called Piper, I was asked to speak and do a demo. It was to be our first. Although extremely nervous, I did my little speech and demonstrated sock removal, dropped phone and keys' retrieval. I now have a bag that I take along to my demonstrations – it didn't do my real mobile any good to be constantly dropped, nor do I necessarily wear socks!

The garage had made a donation for every puncture repaired and every tyre replaced, plus they held various fundraising activities such as this. Later I discovered that there had been a lady with newly diagnosed MS in the audience: always someone will benefit from hearing about our experiences if we just let them be heard. Again, Harmony was fantastic – I even got her to pull the raffle tickets.

Earlier that year, in April, I was asked to attend a fundraising lunch at an exclusive golf club in East Lothian. I decided to take Melissa along as it was during the holidays and I had no one to help me with her that day; Clara came, too. On the journey there, I had tentatively asked Melissa if she would speak and what she might say; together we had practised in the car. It's an annual event: people pay for a ticket, which includes an outdoor demonstration, lunch and a day of golf. We were to speak at the end of the demonstration lead by Andy and various dogs-in-training to show off their abilities. All I could think was: *Help, they have it all covered – and so slickly, too! Now what do I do?* Quietly I passed a piece of cheese to Clara, making sure Harmony saw. I started off slowly by dropping my keys, but explained how essential that task is. Then I sent Harmony into the crowd to find Clara, who had gone on ahead.

After the demonstration, Melissa seemed very relaxed. Having glanced at her, I decided that she could cope. I then crossed my fingers and took a deep breath before announcing: 'I'd like to introduce Melissa.'

She stood up.

'Now talk to the ladies and gentlemen in a big voice,' I whispered encouragingly.

She didn't hesitate.

'Harmony helps my mummy because her legs don't work and she helps me because when I get scared, I can put my face on her and when I am sad, she makes me happy!'

As she sat down, I put my arms around her and gave her the biggest hug a mum could give. No wonder Canine Partners' fundraisers call us 'Team Hyder'.

'Well done, darling,' I told her. 'That was lovely!'

18

By Royal Invitation

It's not every day that a man in a top hat asks if you would like to present your dog to the Queen. As you can imagine, the invitation to attend the Royal Garden Party at Holyrood Palace in July (a far more intimate affair than Buckingham Palace, I'm reliably informed), courtesy of Canine Partners, triggered a major wardrobe crisis. What does one wear to tea with the Queen?

'Don't worry,' said Clara. 'Maxi dresses are in. You'll look fab!'

Isn't it great that long dresses are back in fashion? The maxi will look so elegant with my new wheelchair, too.

Dress bought, all I needed now was a jacket and matching accessories. Mid-week, Clara and I headed down to Princes Street by bus: I was keen to use my big, properly supportive wheelchair and I wanted to go on a bus. I hadn't been on one for years but all the Lothian Regional Transport (LRT) buses now have disabled access. It felt strange not having Harmony at my side, but I also knew she was better off at home – she wouldn't have wanted to be dragged around the shops for hours. Instead I had Clara, my personal shopper.

That first bus ride was so exciting: the ramp came down and it was easy to get on.

'*Mum*, it's just a bus!' Clara protested, as I chatted away excitedly.

First stop was the House of Fraser to look for a jacket. Disability access? Hah! Now believe me, I've been to a lot of places where they don't have wheelchair access. If someone tells me, 'Sorry, we don't have disabled access,' I'll show up in my wheelchair and forcibly introduce it, much to my family's horror. The House of Fraser is old, with all sorts of half-levels. Obviously, I couldn't get to the lift. I had visions of bumping into a purple-rinsed Mrs Slocombe from *Are you being Served?* Now *she* would have saved me! In the end we had to go to a side entrance, where a security guard met me and put a ramp in place. Then it was into the lift and out, only to find the jacket section was on another half-floor.

OK, so off we set through the lingerie section to the disabled lift, except this time the racks were too close together. Bras and pants trailed from my footplates. Clara sighed but put them back.

Into the lift and down we went: no problem. Out of the lift, we found ourselves in an ocean of jackets on sale (*yes!*). It wasn't too long before we had picked out six to try on. So where was the changing room? On the half-level up! So back into the lift and up we went; that's when we hit the really *BIG* problem – the lift had a front entry but a side exit. I'd reversed into the lift on the way up and now I was stuck, totally stuck; I couldn't move forward or backwards. Turning non-existent circles, I could feel the panic rise and tears pricking my eyes.

I HATE THIS LIFE!

I hate the stupidity of engineers and architects who adapt buildings for people like me, but haven't tried them out properly to see if they really work.

YOUR STUPID LIFTS DON'T WORK!

'Mum, *Mum*, calm down! We can work it out.'

My beautiful, brainy daughter was there, telling me to take a deep breath. She handed the jackets to the sales assistant, got down on the floor, removed my head support, squeezed over and took off the foot-plates, leaving my legs trailing. Finally there was just enough room for me to get out. She helped me into the changing room. Another first! This being that the disabled changing room was not doubled up as storage for boxes. We shut the door, Clara gave me a huge cuddle and she helped me to try on the dress we had brought with us.

'*Mum*, you've got the wrong bra on!'

Damn! I had bought some bust scaffolding especially to make me look more elegant but in all the excitement, I'd forgotten to wear it.

'Never mind,' said my ever-patient daughter with a big sigh. 'We can imagine what the dress will look like with the bra you're wearing.'

Then we tried the jackets and began to giggle for some of them looked like something my dad might have worn and literally draped around my shoulders. 'Boyfriend jackets' is how Clara described them. Others were too fussy, badly tailored or just plain silly. In the end, it came down to two: one pink that I loved (it fitted beautifully) and the other was an elegant emerald. I compared prices: the pink was £100 more expensive.

'OK, Clara, we're going green!'

Success. In the meantime the sales assistant had brought over the duty manager. Before I paid, I took her over to the lift, collecting more lingerie on my footplates en route and showed her the problems. She was very pleasant and extremely apologetic, promising to move the racks (of course, she couldn't do anything about the lift itself).

Back down on the ground floor, we got to the side door only to discover the ramp had been moved. Clara went off in search of a security guard and came back with the same man as last time: he didn't have a clue where the ramp was. Eventually a senior sales person appeared; he got the ramp out and I got out of the shop.

OK, so I can shop but not without my lovely daughter, who yet again had to ask for assistance, even crawl across the floor. Feeling more than slightly frazzled, I suggested we took lunch.

'I'll just pop to the loo,' I said.

Great, there was a disabled loo but it had a heavy door that was locked. Someone went to get the key from the bar. In I went. Phew! Ah, now the door was too heavy to open: I couldn't get out. So, I phoned Clara. No reply. Eek! Now I was beginning to panic. OK, reverse chair; now use said chair as a battering ram. Oomph, out!

The rest of the day was relatively simple in terms of wheelchair access and very successful for shopping, too: I found a hat, bag and shoes and jewellery, all in the sales (Clara has an eye for a bargain). As usual, the counters were too high for me to reach and the pin machines couldn't be tilted to facilitate my reading of the screen.

Clara spent the next two days sewing green beads into the necklace, earrings and handbag.

'This way, we can tie your whole outfit together,' she explained.

The great day arrived and it was sunny and warm. I spent the morning horizontal, resting so that I wasn't too tired to enjoy the afternoon. How absurdly cool it felt to drive into a barricaded Holyrood Park, waved through by the police and escorted into a special area for disabled parking. Andrew and I joined the queue, presented our passes and proof of identity and then we were ushered in. The tea tent was stunning with beautiful floral displays; its theme was pink, so there were beautiful cakes and tarts, all pink, tiny sandwiches and large tea urns. The tea wasn't very warm, though: tea from an urn is *still* the same, even from a gold-plated one! Like statues, the Royal Company of Archers stood to attention in their feathers throughout the proceedings, which unsettled Harmony, who began to growl. I gave her a reassuring cuddle.

Oh no, please don't disgrace us now!

So there we were, Andrew and I, nibbling Victoria sponge and drinking (lukewarm) tea with Harmony by our side, watching the Queen chat to those lucky enough to have been plucked from the crowds when out he popped, the man in the top hat! And if he was the Mad Hatter, I must have been Alice.

'Would you care to present your dog to the Queen?' he asked.

'Oh yes, please,' I gasped. 'And can I bring my husband?'

We were ushered through the thousand or so to the inner court, a grassy area where HM Queen Elizabeth stood in a dazzling lilac coat and hat, surrounded by courtiers minus her corgis. She certainly didn't look her age, nor did she seem frail. I couldn't curtsy, so I tipped my head. She smiled at me.

'What's her name?' she asked.

'Harmony.'

'What does she do for you?'

'She takes my laundry out of the washing machine ...'

'Can she undress you?'

'Yes,' I said. 'She's very tidy – she doesn't leave the clothes on the floor. She puts them in my lap for me to put away.'

'Why, every teenager in the country needs a Harmony,' remarked the Queen.

I couldn't have put it better myself.

The sun shone and I'd shared a joke with Her Majesty, who patted Harmony with a gloved hand. What a perfect day. Then, like Alice, I woke up ...

19

Tasting Freedom

Ben Nevis is the highest mountain in the British Isles. The first time I climbed it was with Andrew and his family just before he started a degree at Reading University. I was still training to be a nurse and I knew I would miss him, so we decided to mark the occasion with a climb. We descended using the so-called interesting shortcut that Andrew and his dad decided upon (Andrew never repeats a walk, it's circular walks only for him). All I remember about the ascent was that it seemed endless: afterwards, we were so exhausted that we were too tired to eat the meal I'd prepared in the flat. I remember going to work the next day with chronic discomfort in my thighs and knees – that pain echoed the feeling in my heart as I began a new life in Edinburgh, alone and without Andrew.

If you're a ropes-and-crampons climber, the main attraction of Ben Nevis is the 700-metre (2,290-feet) north-facing cliffs. The pony track is the easiest route up and was originally constructed to enable ponies to take supplies to the staff manning the Victorian observatory at the top. As you can imagine, it was the perfect spot for meteorology readings. Ben Nevis also plays its part in Scottish mythology but that's another story.

Knowing my hill-climbing days were over, when did I decide to have another appointment with Scotland's Everest? I'd have to be honest and say it was in response to a request from Canine Partners.

Here I need to rewind to one Monday morning in February when the phone rang.

'Sally. Good morning, it's Annemarie [the then Scottish fundraiser for Canine Partners] here. We're organising a new press campaign for 2010 and would love to photograph you and Harmony. Can you think of somewhere iconic and Scottish?'

'Lots of things come to mind. Can I have a think about it and get back to you?' I asked.

Immediately, I set my mind to thinking about it. Edinburgh Castle? A bit obvious, perhaps. Scottish Parliament? Boring and ugly! Mountains, hills, lochs … Ben Nevis … How cool was that? A picture of Harmony and me at the top of Ben Nevis! I wish …

As soon as Ben Nevis crossed my radar, that was it: I began wondering if there was any way that Harmony and I could get to the top. I googled all-terrain vehicles before mentally discarding them all as unsuitable for what I had in mind.

In 2009, the NHS had reassessed me for an electric wheelchair. They tried hard to prove that I wasn't sufficiently disabled to qualify but in the end I was deemed 'bad enough'. After this, they were incredibly helpful and supportive: they allocated me a chair to accommodate my spasms and inability to sit up straight. I can tilt in space (i.e. I keep sitting) but the chair tilts backwards and so rather than recline (which stretches my legs and back), this keeps my legs bent in the normal sitting position but takes the pain out of my back and doesn't put me in a spasm (which an ordinary recliner does). But, and it's a very big but, the NHS outdoor wheelchair will only go on tarmac.

As I have already mentioned, my scooter took me to places it shouldn't have done when I was out exercising Harmony, but I wanted more. Hurrah, I had found it! An off-road wheelchair that would endure 16 kilometres of rocky terrain to reach the summit and get me safely back again; it's called the Boma and is made by Molten Rock, who are based in Milton Keynes (the chair was invented by sports enthusiast, Chris Swift, who has been a tetraplegic since the age of 19). It looked perfect; it looked *fantastic*! Orange, with thick mountain-bike tyres, the chair embodied the outdoor spirit of disabled people such as Chris and me.

Mountain bike-orientated technology means the Boma can go upstairs and downstairs (the website had pictures to prove it – it had been tested in Africa and the Alps). It's portable and operates with handlebars similar to those of a motorbike. I read how someone had travelled all the way from East to West across England on a Boma. It looked like a cross between two mountain bikes put together and a go-kart. I wanted one: at the very least, I was eager to try one.

First of all, I had to ring Annemarie.

'Hi, Sally here,' I said. 'So, OK, how about doing the photo-shoot at the top of Ben Nevis? I'm thinking that I could do it as a fundraiser for Canine Partners as well.'

At first, I was met by stunned silence at the other end.

'*Right.* So, how are you going to do that?' she eventually asked.

I explained about Molten Rock.

'Just leave it to me,' she said, and promptly rang Molten Rock and got through to Chris.

'Don't think of it as a wheelchair,' advised Chris, after she had tracked him down. 'Think of it as a four-wheel mountain bike.'

Chris couldn't have been friendlier or more eager to help in any way he could. Indeed, he agreed to lend me a Boma for the climb itself and also for training. Two months later, Stuart (the company's Scottish rep) brought one down. I felt like a pioneer – I'd never imagined it was possible to feel so brave and intrepid, to be in the position of taking a giant step for womankind. Indeed, I was grinning from ear to ear. I didn't think of the Boma as a wheelchair; I didn't have any of the residual sadness I feel when I'm getting into my regular wheelchair. Instead, as I lowered myself into the bucket seat with its low centre of gravity, I was mentally attaching the mountain bikes to the back of the car and taking off for a day's adventuring! Stuart showed me how to use the controls (basically the Boma is operated by two dry-cell batteries that sit in front). I got in and discovered that even the handlebars move to accommodate legs that can't lift over, switched it on and off we went. Harmony had to trot to keep up with us.

'It's so comfy,' I kept saying. 'It's so fast.'

In contrast to the jerky, stop-start experience of using a wheelchair, this was an incredibly smooth ride. I had an immediate sense of speed. Suddenly I could go *anywhere*, my horizons were no longer confined. I kicked it into full power and off I went.

Chris left it with us. Five days later, Andrew and I drove up into the Pentland Hills for the first time in almost a decade. It felt *so* good! Harmony took one look at me and came over as if to say: *Shall we?* I recognised the look in her eyes. *Come on, I dare you – give it some Wellie!* I opened the throttle and we flew around the field in ways I'd only ever dreamed of. Harmony ran with me, ears back, fur flying.

'It's just like the old days,' said Andrew with a huge grin. 'I've even got muddy boots!'

Melissa was on respite and so it was just the two of us, the hearty walkers of old. Life felt real: we weren't on a disability track and I didn't have to worry about tree roots or dropped kerbs. The wind was blowing and the air was fresh. We made our way along the road and then turned off onto the path beside a stream. The sun twinkled on the water like diamonds. Already, I was doing something my soul had been yearning for. We kept going: over the bridge, up the stone steps, up a steep incline and onto the hillside. I started squealing, it was scary.

But the Boma didn't tilt: it careered across the uneven ground, with me in it. Harmony splashed in the stream and charged over the hill. She kept coming back to check I was OK. We approached the top but I wasn't confident enough to try the really steep bit. I cut the engine and we sat in silence and looked out at the view.

A walker, coming from the opposite direction, stopped in his tracks and stared. There was a sharp intake of breath.

'How the fuck did you get up here?' he asked.

I laughed: it felt great to be part of the walking community again, to be back in the hills. I'd forgotten how many smiles and nods you get; how many people you meet with a common goal. We headed back down and stopped at the pub with our muddy dog. I had the best pint I've ever drunk: the sense of freedom and exhilaration was incredible. Harmony had spurred us on to this wonderful moment. Perhaps with the Boma I could once more see the top of a Munro?

This was what Harmony had given me: she had inspired me to start enjoying the outdoors again. Despite my accident in the woodlands earlier that year when I slipped on the ice, I felt safe wherever I went with Harmony by my side.

'I think I might get my mountain bike out again,' mused Andrew.

And it wasn't just me who had Harmony to thank: the whole family's spirit of adventure had been restored. The following weekend we drove to Glentress, a forest near Peebles in the south of Scotland. It was a place where we had often walked as a family and even held a birthday party for Peter there. Ten boys, each armed with a water pistol, battled in teams (refuelling at the Lochen). Happy memories! So back we went. The place has become a Mecca for mountain-bike riders – there are lots of mountain-bike trails. Andrew walked and I was in the Boma; we met bikers coming the other way, who were genuinely impressed by my vehicle.

'Now that's a cool piece of kit!'

I was thrilled. Not only was my disability invisible but now I was scoring brownie points for my kit, too. Way to go!

The July weekend of the trial run up Ben Nevis arrived. At the last minute Chris Swift and Jon, the company engineer, rang to say they couldn't make it (Chris's car was in the garage and Jon was overwhelmed with work). It was huge disappointment: I wanted them to see 'the Ben', as we call it here in Scotland, and meet Andrew but I knew how hard they work and what a mammoth undertaking it was, getting to Edinburgh. However, they sent spare batteries and fuses up on an overnight courier and Jon spoke to Andrew to explain how to change the fuses.

Preparations involved packing for an overnight stay and I had to make sure I had all Harmony's gear and mine. Paramo, an outdoor gear company, lent me three pairs of amazing trousers plus jackets to keep me warm and dry. We (that's me with Andrew, Peter, his girlfriend, Clara and Melissa) finally set off at 11am and arrived an hour late (caravans in Scotland in the summer, groan!). We travelled in two cars, as we also had the Boma. We arrived at the bunkhouse accommodation owned by Alan, the mountain guide we had engaged for the attempt (he's a lovely man with a weather-beaten face and twinkling eyes). While hugely supportive of our expedition, he was also something of a doubting Thomas, though.

'This is the machine, huh?' He looked doubtfully over towards the Boma. 'Are you happy to get on with it?'

'Yes,' I said, excited but nervous too.

'Well, let's go.'

We threw on our walking gear and followed Alan, who has lived in Fort William for 40 years. What he doesn't know about Ben Nevis and the surrounding mountains can be written on a postage stamp (he also guides in the Alps and other mountains); we were hugely lucky to have him with his love for, and knowledge of, mountains. We drove to the base and parked by the Ben Nevis Inn, the main resting point after a walk. It's s simple wooden structure with a ramp leading to the top floor, where the bar is located – now that's what I call 'access all areas'!

Jacqui, a local physiotherapist, and Stuart, the Scottish Boma rep, were waiting for us at the Inn.

'I'm impressed by this machine,' said Alan, who was obviously coming round to it, as Andrew and Stuart got talking about the Boma. Meanwhile, I had to curb my impatience: I wanted to get up that mountain.

'Great day for it,' continued Alan. 'Unusually there is no rain. We were forecast gales and rain. We're lucky – the weather's on our side.'

Lucky indeed … Boots on, kit on. Off we went.

Tasting Freedom

Even Melissa wanted to try walking some of the way. With her hand trustingly in Clara's, she stepped onto her first mountain and up we went. Peter's girlfriend had Harmony on the lead (the early part of the Ben is grazing and we didn't want her to chase the sheep). Dogs should always be kept on the lead around sheep and I am sure that given the chance, Harmony – just like any other young dog – would succumb to temptation and enjoy chasing them. We came to our first obstacle: a stile with a locked gate to the side. Out I got and the team lifted the Boma over it. Peter hauled me over the stile as Alan remarked, 'We'll get the key to the gate for the ascent.'

'Can someone make a note of that?' I asked.

Off we went. (Note to self: When someone says there are great big boulders and stone steps to clamber over, don't dismiss it. Believe them.)

'Go for it!' everyone said, and so I did and the Boma made it … so far.

We encountered the first of the drainage ditches designed to channel the water off the mountain and ensure the path doesn't become eroded. These ditches have large slabs of rock either side with a 10-inch gap in the middle. *Easy*, I thought as I went whizzing over the gap. Then came the next slab.

'Can't I go round it?' I asked Alan.

'No,' came his stern reply. 'You must stick to the path!'

He was right, of course: only by sticking to the path will we conserve the Ben and its wilderness. This time we had someone behind me and someone else either side of me in case I tipped out. But I didn't and so on we went.

Each time we stopped, Melissa (still clutching her big sister's hand) caught up with us. It was a miracle: she was climbing up and up until, as expected, eventually she had had enough and Clara kindly took her back down again. Unfortunately, Melissa slipped and fell, which resulted in Clara having to manage a panic attack. But she did it – well done, Big Sis!

My attempts to negotiate the difficult terrain made Harmony very uneasy, however: she was barking and whining. If she was off the lead, she was fine because she could stay near me. On the lead, it was very hard for her. Every time we stopped, she came up to me as if to nag and grumble and checked me all over. It seemed to be easier if she was ahead so long as she knew I was OK and on my way.

We crossed more stone outcrops. This was not the smooth track of my childhood, or had I failed to notice the tricky bits when my legs were working? As we went up and over another outcrop, the steering twisted out of my hand. I banged a rear wheel on a rock, squashing Jacqui and Peter and running over Andrew's foot. We came to a standstill. Well, that's one way to end an expedition: knock everyone else off the mountain with your vehicle.

'Is everyone OK?' I asked.

There was a chorus of ayes, then on we went: I was getting higher and the houses were beginning to look tiny. For the first time in years, I was getting a view.

BANG!

'Stop!' everyone shouted. 'What's happened?'

'Oh dear!'

Disaster, the rear wheel had come off. Stuart, who initially had no intention of coming up the mountain, was luckily on hand. Off I got with Harmony all over me: licking, checking that I was OK. Her concerns had been legitimate; she circled me with a look of pity and indignation: *Now you've done it, Sally! You've really done something stupid, haven't you?* While emergency repairs were undertaken, I sat on the ground and gazed down on Glen Nevis: it looked so green and serene, the toy houses and cars blinking in the sun. Was this it? Would I have to call a halt to the Big Adventure?

'That should do it,' said Stuart.

The wheel went on, but we decided to descend: in total, we had covered under two kilometres. Although heartbroken and deeply disappointed, I was trying hard not to show how I felt. It was a quieter group on the way down: this time ropes were attached to the back of the Boma in case of emergency where it would be necessary to lower me down the rocky outcrops. The descent was well managed and we made fast progress, although the wheel once more came off.

Back at base, we marked the end of our trial run with a round of drinks at the Ben Nevis Inn. Jacqui's little boy, who was only four, came up to meet us with his dad. He told us that his father looked after him when Mum was out at work.

'What do you do with Daddy?' I asked.

'Skiing and bouldering and stuff,' he said.

What a cool dad and what a great life!

That night, after a fish and chip supper we chattered about the day and Peter was great.

'We'd just got complacent because the Boma was doing so well,' he insisted. 'If we really avoid each major obstacle then we will manage it – Mum, you *will* get to the top!'

Tired and sore, I retired to bed in the bunkhouse, but with Peter's encouraging words ringing in my ears: I didn't know what to do – should I make the attempt? I felt overwhelmed with gratitude that my family had all come up to support me. The next morning, we had a meeting with Alan.

'What about doing a different Munro with an easier track?' he suggested. 'Otherwise, if they can beef up the Boma, we'll be with you if you want to do the Ben.'

'I'd rather try and fail the Ben than dumb down the challenge,' I said, after a deep breath. After all, I had to be true to myself.

'Let's go for it!' said Alan.

The family cheered: at that moment, I was so proud of my ruddy-faced lot for encouraging their mum to complete the task with Harmony. It made me feel enormously happy and confident. Andrew beamed at me. The real challenge would be the August climb: this would be our Everest.

'You wouldn't want it to be any easier, would you?' said Andrew.

A few days later I received an email from Alan. Jacqui, the physiotherapist, had been talking to someone at the John Muir Trust (a charity that owns and manages lots of

Scotland's open spaces) about the challenge and she suggested going onto Ben Nevis via a different route, one the quad bikes had been using while upgrading the path. The route still had markers and they would leave them there until after I had completed the challenge. There was a minor problem of a river to cross and it was slightly further, but it met the track about halfway up and so reduced the enormous rocks by 50 per cent. It sounded better and it was unusual too.

Excellent, full steam ahead then!

20

Finishing on a High

On 17 August 2010, I received some bad news: one of my main teams (consisting of eight) had pulled out. The couple that built this particular team had some terrible news: the woman's mother had died unexpectedly, 17 weeks after her father passed away. Of course, it was devastating for them and I shared their sorrow; I was also upset to lose two key members from the team.

I phoned Giorgio, owner of Stobhan (the B&B that the team were booked into). He was fantastic and said not to worry. Afterwards, I emailed everyone to make sure I had their consent forms and menu choices. I still needed to do a schedule for the weekend.

By 23 August, one of my main concerns was that I hadn't been on the Boma since the trial – Stuart had been too busy to get it back to me, fixed. There was a definite knack to managing the machine and I hoped I hadn't forgotten how; also, we had never done a serious climb while training without the engine overheating and cutting out but at least we now knew that we had to give it time to rest and I couldn't hold it back to go at a walking pace as that would compound the problem. I wasn't scared of an accident but would my body hold up or go into a massive spasm? Already, I'd taken double the dosage of my anti-spasm drugs and had brought more with me. In the park, all my dog-walking friends wished me well for the mad venture. Without the Boma, I would need Andrew to take Harmony on extra runs to maintain her fitness levels.

In retrospect, perhaps I should have allowed someone else to do the admin for the event. I just felt so touched and excited that people were behind it and I didn't want to add to their burden. Now I was having sleepless nights and wondering whether I'd covered everything.

By 25 August, the nerves really were settling in: I was so scared of failure. It wasn't an option as far as I was concerned, but it might happen – I had to be realistic. I wasn't sure how I'd feel if this proved to be the case; I'd just have to wait and see. Meanwhile, *The Hour* and STV News had been in touch, asking to cover the story. As always, it was a 'maybe' so once again, we would need to be patient. At the same time, a friend shared the Just Giving website with all his friends on Facebook and suddenly, my own Just Giving site took off all over again.

I couldn't help but feel a bit sad at this point that I wouldn't be able to raise all the money that I wanted to, but we had certainly raised the profile of Canine Partners. Also, I was really looking forward to seeing everyone at the weekend.

On 27 August, I was texted to say that someone with MS but ambulant (someone walking, not using a wheelchair or aids) had just failed to reach the summit. I really could have done without knowing that. I spent an hour coordinating the food for Saturday – the level of organisation was really driving me crazy by then; I was glad to hand it all over to Andrew and just hoped he would understand my cryptic notes.

At this point I hadn't heard back from STV News or *The Hour* and so I assumed it wasn't going to happen. Onwards and upwards.

With butterflies in my stomach, we set off at 9am on Saturday, 28 August. Mandy, a friend from London, accompanied us there. The bunkhouses, owned by Alan our mountain guide, were just perfect: more like flatlets than shared dorms, they are so comfortable. Even their name – 'Calluna', which is Latin for the mountain heather that grows everywhere – is pretty. All but one family had arrived. Alan briefed everyone: yes, it might be August but there's still a foul weather warning with the possibility of snow.

Meatballs, pasta and wine all round were followed by birthday cake for Elaine (one of the trainers). We finally threw everyone out at 9pm so that we could get to bed. Even so, I couldn't sleep: I was so scared of failure. The mountaintop looked incredibly high and while I'd been to the top before, I'd never done so in a wheelchair. (Note to self: next time you have a good idea, take a tot of whisky and lie down – then keep it to yourself!) However, there was a happy end to the day for Melissa climbed her own Ben Nevis: she went up Blackford Hill in Edinburgh – a pretty big climb for someone like her. She walked up it with Ali (who had come to look after her while I was on my big adventure) and Megan, one of her school friends. She was so proud to have got there – and I was a proud mum!

Talking of proud mums, my own had arrived the day before and was soon ensconced in her room. We arrived to find her happily dispensing mugs of tea all round. Dad had stayed home – no way would his knees allow for Ben Nevis. I chatted happily with Chris, who had arrived with the Boma. It meant a lot to me that Mum was there; my in-laws, Rob and Delia, also came along to provide invaluable moral and practical support. They served meatballs and pasta to 40 people and for me, their presence was a huge boost.

Finally, Ben Nevis Day: 29 August. Overnight there had been strong winds and torrential rain but the morning looked clear and beautiful, with blue skies and no wind. We were off in the car to join the other members of Team A for a 7am start.

Stepping out of the bunkhouse door, I notice Tibetan prayer flags fluttering in the breeze: it's a beautiful moment of symmetry with Everest all those years ago and fills me with hope. Even the muted blues and oranges and the Tibetan writing are the same; they look as if they've been here forever. I ask Alan where they came from: he tells me that he brought them back from a trip to Nepal. I send up a prayer of my own. In the Old Testament, Nehemiah finds himself in a very tricky situation and sends up 'a prayer like an arrow' (straight to God). I too like 'arrow prayers' and this was one such moment.

Keep everyone safe, please and help me get up there.

It's difficult to move: I am wrapped in so many layers of equipment that I'm unable to bend in the middle (not that bending is my forte these days!). At the same time, I'm so warm that I have everything vented and unzipped as much as possible – I get grumpy when I'm too hot.

At the car park, we meet the guides from West Coast Mountain Guides and the rest of Team A – that's Jacqui, Alan and Nick plus all the trainers from Canine Partners: Vicky, Elaine, Claire, Anna, Ann, Gemma, Laura, Ronnie and Gemma's boyfriend, Matt. Then there's Peter, his girl-friend and their friend Amy, Andrew and Jon, the engineer for the Boma. Jon's backpack looks huge – he says he has enough kit in there to rebuild the Boma and it certainly appears heavy. Clare and Andy are there, too: they are media students working on their Masters portfolio who will be doing the filming and photography. We also managed to find volunteers to carry the batteries: there are 10 extra batteries and each one weighs 6.5kg (14lb 5oz).

One has already gone up with Team B; Peter and the girls take two. Mandy has one, Andrew has another and Jon adds one to his full rucksack. I hand Harmony over to Ann.

Where are you going?

'Don't worry,' I tell Harmony. 'I'm right here!'

Ronnie is looking after their dog, Erin. Other dogs include Enya, an enormous shy creature of mixed parentage, Pig, a Staffie (whose low body means not a lot of clearance for the rocks on Ben Nevis) and Doyle, my old friend from Canine Partners. All the dogs feast on banana and porridge for energy (breakfast for Olympians) and are put on leads to preserve their power; also out of respect for any livestock we might come across.

'Morning, team!'

'All set?'

'Here we go!'

Encouraged by happy banter as we set off, I'm nevertheless anxious about the Boma's ability to cope: will my body stay upright for that length of time? I keep my anxieties to myself.

The track is relatively easy: it's the quad bike track. I let my guard down and start to enjoy myself. I mean, I might as well, right? After all, that's what it's all about. I'm reminded of hill walking as a little girl and feel the pit of dread I had in the car recede as I give in to the rhythm, taking one step at a time; I can hear my breath. Already I feel a sense of achievement, knowing that it's a Forestry Commission trail heading to the North Face (the very dangerous face mountaineers climb). I feel cool being part of a gang, doing a real climb.

At first we go through the woods. The plan is to circle round and meet the main path at the halfway point. Once again, a passing mountaineer sees the Boma and comes over to check it out.

'Cool! Awesome kit – I could do with one of those.'

I love the fact that they don't see me or my disability just the kit.

Up we go! The Boma's in fine fettle and I find myself leaving everyone behind as I motor up the track. Every now and again I have to stop at a particularly steep part. Andrew walks as close to me as he can; there's no room for anyone next to me: people are walking in twos. Harmony doesn't like being apart and takes every opportunity to check up on me, give me a lick and tell me off.

Oh no, not another stop!

The engine has overheated and when this happens the Boma shuts down so I have to bang on the brake and wait it out. But it's not a problem: we were prepared for such an eventuality and know how to resolve it: just sit and wait for the Boma to cool down.

'You keep going,' I tell the trainers and Mum.

Andrew and Jon stay with me, as does Jacqui. I'll soon catch the others up. Harmony is with Ann and my poor dog has no idea what I'm doing or why she's on the lead when we're in the middle of woods.

'It's OK, Harmony, go with Ann!' I tell her. 'I will catch up soon.'

Ann gets her part of the way up but then Harmony decides to hold a sitting protest. She sits down and clenches her muscles, refusing to go another inch until I'm on the move again.

While I wait, I look up: above in a narrow gap between the trees, I can see blue sky.

The sky's the limit, Sally!

Finishing on a High

The scent of pine fills my lungs as I watch Harmony sniff in the direction of wild deer and rodents lurking somewhere in the woods. The engine starts and off we go again. Now the climb gets steeper but it's manageable and I still feel warm in my padding. The path ends and gosh, it's a car park!

'What, do you mean we could have started from here?'

Oh well, so that was just the warm-up, the dry run and here comes the real climb. I'm feeling bullish. We cross the car park.

'Come on, no hanging around, let's go!' I order the troops.

'Hang on, Sally! We're just checking the river is low enough for you to get across,' says Alan.

Beyond the car park the path declines steeply to a river. We can hear gurgling water and feel the cool, damp air.

'I brought planks up here yesterday,' Alan tells me. 'To help you with your entry.'

The river is roughly twenty feet wide with fast, rushing water. Ferns curl towards the water's edge, flanked by tiny pebble beaches. One by one, the team walks across a very thin pole, clutching a hand-height wire fence. Peter guides everyone across, taking rucksacks and generally lending encouragement. At this point, I realise I'm missing Clara dreadfully – she has had to stay behind to attend a scout training camp.

I make my way down Alan's planks, enter the river and aim for the landing point on the other side. Engine in full throttle, I drive upstream, landing safely to applause from the other side. That was so much fun splashing through the water! The dogs need to be encouraged to the other side. With wagging tails, they make it after having had a good drink en route.

'Now here's that bit of bog I told you about,' says Alan.

Bit? All I can see is purple: the heather and myrtle bog go on forever. No track. Squinting, we can just make out the old quad bike tracks. Alan decides the best way to cross is to go alongside the track. We set off with everyone sprinting alongside me, parting the heather to make way for the Boma. Harmony has disappeared into the undergrowth, head down, as she follows the multitude of smells.

But then the engine cuts out once. Twice. Three times. Every time I hear it splutter, my heart misses a beat, my stomach lurches. I will the Boma not to give up and offer up a silent prayer.

Come on, girl – you can do it!

'This bog is really straining her,' says Jon, the saintly engineer with the heavy rucksack of parts on his back.

He makes the executive decision to switch off the Boma: the engine needs to cool down. We have to stop for a bit. Each time the engine overheats it takes a good 10 minutes to cool off enough to let it go again.

While we wait, the team admire the scenery. At this height we've got a bird's-eye view of the rivers and lochs threading their way across the green valley like silver on an emerald brooch. Already I'm silently celebrating the fact that I'm actually higher than I've been in a long time.

'It looks like the battery has gone,' says Jon, looking up from the front of the Boma.

'Do you know something, Jon?' I reply. 'I'm beginning to *hate* batteries!'

He laughs. Laughter soon fades to sighs of irritation as two replacement batteries are fitted; each time Jon tries the engine only to discover they won't start. Both have run out.

Not good! We're going through them so fast that at this rate I won't … But I refuse to allow myself to finish that thought.

'I carried it all this way and it's **** empty!' Peter curses.

'How many fresh batteries does Team B have with them?' I ask.

'Only one,' says Jon. 'This is odd – one is empty and the other is full.'

So, we're down to four batteries. Jon replaces the duds with two of the last remaining four. The engine starts and the Boma carries me up and down through the heather.

'Look,' suddenly Ann calls a halt. Far below and across the loch is the tallest, brightest rainbow I've ever seen. God's promise, *I will never leave you*, springs to mind. I allow myself to believe anything is possible. The Boma is struggling so much that, in order to preserve battery power, it's decided ropes will be attached to it. Jon, Alan and Andrew tie them to cleats, which were put onto the Boma for exactly this reason. I steer as I'm pushed and pulled and the engines rev. Everyone now jogs with me, running to get on ahead and then relaying to push me: I feel like a Victorian explorer carried by Sherpas. Everyone is helping, wielding heavy loads and looking exhausted; they are all slipping and sliding, trying to keep themselves and me upright.

Too late! Suddenly the Boma tips and out I fall like a sack of potatoes. I'm not hurt – the bog and heather make for a soft landing – however, I am stuck. Someone's hand reaches in and undoes the safety strap; people are pulling me out. Harmony barks and runs between people's legs. All I can see are walking boots.

'Stop,' I call out. 'My leg!'

My leg is caught in the Boma and won't bend. Eventually I'm extricated and I start to laugh. I look over at the camera team: 'Please tell me you got that on film.'

But they shake their heads: they were too busy trying to rescue me. Ah well, it would have made great telly. Aren't all comedies tragedies in disguise?

'Well, don't ask for a Take Two!' I tell them.

Finally I'm back in the Boma, waterproofs and clothing rearranged, legs intact. Harmony is now calm and in front of us, we see the main path.

'Afternoon!'

It's Team B.

'Fresh blood!' goes up the cry from an exhausted Team A.

Alan tells everyone to take a good break. Besides, it's time for lunch – we've been climbing for a good four hours. We need, we *deserve* a break. Everyone flops down in the heather and digs out their sandwiches and flasks. Team B consists of Debbie and Jane (friends of mine),

Mark and Fiona (friends of Andrew), Harmony's puppy parent Lesley and her daughter plus another puppy parent, Alison. Finally, there's a dad and his two sons aged 12 and 15 – kind volunteers who have been walking up the main route and set off at 9am. Good timing: as planned, we've all met at the halfway Lochen. Team B's guides, Jamie and Richard, have done a fantastic job as has everyone else.

Peter has carried so many people's rucksacks – he hasn't stopped pulling or pushing all day, while making sure everyone has been OK. I couldn't have asked for a better mountain guide.

'Mum, have you eaten that Boost I gave you?' he shouts.

Everyone laughs.

Busted! I've secretly snacked on chocolate to get me up the mountain.

'Come on, folks,' Alan tells us. 'Time to move on!'

Everyone seems happy: they're loving the views. Some have never been to Scotland or climbed a mountain before; the weather is just fantastic and the lower mountains look good. I feel so proud of my home country as I see them all enjoying it. Harmony has a great cuddle, a banana for energy and a drink.

Alan takes charge, saying: 'No time to waste! We've got another four hours of climbing.'

We set off again and this time Teams A and B are united; that means 28 walkers plus dogs, guides and me. Apart from the drainage channels that are chasms across the track (oh so easy to fall into one of those), the track feels wonderfully easy after the bog; I'm confident. I've no idea of the time – it all seems to be going so quickly – but I'm feeling sore and tired so I know we've been going for hours. The track has been evened out with gravel to facilitate the huge number of people who use it (Alan reckons about 1,000 over the weekend); it's one way to try and prevent the mountain from being eroded. Everyone must stick to the path and there are also signs asking folk to keep dogs on leads to prevent accidents.

I'm beginning to recognise the Boma's 'I'm tired' signals. Sure enough, after a few flashing lights the engine cuts out and a fresh battery (carried by Team B) is produced. It's the last change: for some reason the batteries seem to be getting weaker. They last for less time or does the ascent as we reach the top mean the Boma needs more power?

Five minutes later, it cuts out.

'Jon, what's going on?'

I sense myself beginning to panic.

The group gathers round and everyone looks apprehensive. As usual, my lovely dog takes the opportunity to give me a cuddle.

Oh Harmony, how I love you!

Jon looks up at me and I can see it in his eyes before he says anything but I don't want to hear what he has to say.

'Sally, it's the circuit board – it's fused. I can put a new one in, but because it's been drawing energy exclusively off one battery, we have used them too quickly. We have lost those two empty ones from the supply. I hate to say it, but we don't have enough batteries to get you to the top.'

Silence.

'We can pull you up the rest of the way, Mum.'

It's Peter, my little soldier, now a young man.

I smile at him; I have to think fast – it's another two hours to get to the top. There's no way I can ask the team to do that, already they look tired. Besides, I wanted to do it under Boma steam. This was supposed to be *my* climb!

'Right,' I say, swallowing back the tears – a mix of anger, disappointment and extreme sadness. 'I'm going back down. The rest of you carry on, get to the top and shout my name.'

No one wants to leave me, so I put on a brave face and force a smile.

'Really,' I insist.

But they don't look at all convinced.

'It's your dream, too – it's what you've been sponsored to do and training to do.'

'Sally …'

'I won't hear any excuses!'

And so the team move off, but Mandy (my good friend and Peter's godmother) refuses to leave me.

'Mandy,' I fix her with one of my looks. 'I need you to go more than I need you to stay! You've tried to go up so many times and always been thwarted by the weather. Conditions are perfect today. *GO!*'

Hugs all round and off she goes. Meanwhile, Lesley (Harmony's puppy parent) is in tears.

'I'm coming down with you,' says Mum, defiant, even though I know this will be a huge disappointment to her.

I burst into tears and cuddle Andrew. I feel so angry and devastated – it hurts! Then I pull myself together. I ask Andrew to text Clara and his parents to let them know as they are waiting for news.

Arms around you, comes straight back in a text from Rob and Delia; it helps a lot.

'Can someone take a photo of Harmony and me here?'

Clare snaps away without asking how I feel; I know she and Andy were filming me while I was upset but I had told them to keep rolling, come what may. The final stragglers, still unwilling to leave, are silent. It's a far cry from the chatter and laughter, endless words of encouragement that had all been such a part of the big day.

We begin our descent.

With me are Andrew, Jacqui, Mum, Claire, Alan and Jon. My bladder, with which I normally have no sensation, is full to bursting; every jolt is painful. Andrew has brought a large sheet with him and finds a likely rock. He, Jacqui and Mum hold it around me. Andrew gets all my layers off: now I'm just wearing my upper layers. Ah, what bliss to be caressed by mountain air, to feel my body in contact with Mother Nature!

'I want to walk on a mountain again before I get back in the chair,' I say.

Andrew supports me and off I go, upright – it feels so good. The track is clear. Triumphant, I keep on walking, forcing my unwilling legs to continue.

Just a bit further, Sally!

'You'll have to bring the Boma to me,' I shout back.

The group brings it down to me. Gemma (one of the trainers) and her boyfriend Matt have joined us. It was too much for her, too (I hope it's not the energy she expended on helping me through the bog that has sapped her). Suddenly my right leg feels terrible: a spasm is starting and my brain won't connect with it and so I can't get it to move. I feel dizzy.

'OK, back into the Boma,' I tell Andrew.

We arrive at the bog and of course, we've no power – we have to do the journey in manual without any downhill control. *All that training to control the descent and now look at us!* Alan and Matt attach ropes to the back and with Jon and Andrew at the front, I ease forward, the ropes serving as brakes. Meanwhile, Doyle and Harmony love their romp through the bracken, barking and chasing frogs; they force me to smile. Then Harmony appears at my side, nodding. She catches my eye as if to say, *Wow, what a great day!*

Harmony knows how to make me feel better – she always does, even though my cherished dream is in tatters. Not only have I been unsuccessful, I've needed all this help too.

'Look!' says Jacqui.

We gaze upwards: the teams should be at the top by now. Suddenly I gasp as the summit appears through the mist. *Wow, the views from the top must be incredible!* A pang of jealousy gives way to a tide of gratitude and pleasure that the others have benefited from this amazing trip. On average, the Ben only reveals itself 50 days per year – and today is one of them.

I'm pulled back across the river. Everyone is in pain and exhausted: this time we're grateful for the top car park. We all sit in the sunshine while Andrew and Alan go down to bring up cars for us plus the ill-fated Boma. We hear that two women, a dog and a man have turned back; I feel sad for them. Vicky has had to turn back as her lovely dog, Enya, developed a limp. Ronnie came down too and Alison's legs simply refused to carry on. Enya, I'm glad to say, turns out to be fine.

Back at the bunkhouse, Andrew changes out of sopping clothes. I want to go and see the others back at base, the Ben Nevis Inn. Family and friends are all waiting. An hour later, the last of our team get in. Pints all round! We greet the returning teams with a round of applause. Half an hour later, the most enormous portions of beefsteak and lasagne are served followed by pudding. The mood is tired, but I'm glad to say, happy: so many people who never dreamt they could do the Ben have achieved the climb. Out of 28 walkers, 23 made it.

Twelve-year-old Peter presents me with a rock – he thought he'd bring the summit to me. My own Peter also gives me a beautiful stone that he too brought down. Again, I cry – I thought I was so in control of my emotions, but obviously not.

Back at the bunkhouse, I find lots of lovely Facebook messages from supporters, encouraging me and telling me how well we have all done. Andrew and I end the day with a cup of tea and a wee whisky. Of course, I can't sleep – the spasms are terrible, my head spins. Harmony jumps up beside me and eventually I drift off.

Next morning, I see the trainers packing up, ready to go. I look up at the glorious mountains: they are stunning in the sunshine. A germ of an idea forms. Jon comes round to see me, clearly disappointed the Boma didn't get me get me to the top.

'Don't apologise,' I tell him. 'You did everything you could. Anyway, I've got an idea …'

I watch a smile creep across his face.

'*Really*, Jon – I think we can do it. I want to try again.'

He doesn't look at all surprised.

'If we get guides to take the batteries up the day before and leave them in strategic points, if the Boma Mark 7 is ready. When the path at the top is finished …'

'OK,' says Jon.

That's all I need to hear.

'2011,' I say.

And so, Ben Nevis 2 is born.

On the drive home with Mandy and Harmony in the back, I feel a rush of excitement. There are so many things to look forward to and I can't wait to see Melissa's smiling face – I always miss her when we're apart and I know how much she worries. My thoughts turn to the future. So what's next? Hey, how about abseiling down the Forth Rail Bridge as a warm-up to Ben Nevis 2? But I'm forgetting Machu Pichu, the Alps. Oh yes, and I want to sail the Caledonian Canal …

Finding Harmony

As I write this, I glance over at Harmony, who is sleeping peacefully. Sensing movement, her eyes open and she looks at me to check if I need anything. She is always thinking of me: if I drop something, she comes running. She'll always be there for me, no matter what. As a family, we're flying: Peter is now at Uni, Clara is incredibly busy with her music and Scouts, Melissa now attends a special school … Life is good. Perhaps we could have had adventures without Harmony, but she has given us all the confidence to try new things.

And as for me: I want to *live* the rest of my life, *not* survive it!

Acknowledgements

Jemima Hunt, without whom this book would never have been born; Mum and Dad for showing me mountains; Viv, you know why, and thank you; Ali, for being the best friend ever; Dean for being fun and the most amazing listener; thanks Clara for the title to chapter 13.

Thank you also to Harmony's Puppy Parents: Lesley, Tanya, Wendy, Kevin and Dizzy, plus the fabulous Southampton Puppy Training Satellite, and not forgetting Ann, Harmony's advanced trainer – Harmony is who she is because of all of you.

Thanks to all the Canine Partners Puppy Parents who work so hard – only to face heartbreak each time they pass one of their charges to Advanced Training; to Canine Partner's amazing band of trainers who match us with such skill, and who cope with training not only the dogs but the human side of the partnership as well – and who do all this with unfailing courtesy and enthusiasm: thanks to Guide Dogs for the Blind, who bred Harmony.

Thanks to every person at the charity Canine Partners, for what they do for all of us; to Jenny for being a sounding board and to Wendy for keeping us on the straight and narrow! Finally: to Chris and Jon of Molten Rock – thanks for that Taste of Freedom.

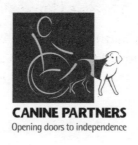

CANINE PARTNERS
Opening doors to independence

Canine Partners

Canine Partners is a registered charity that assists people with disabilities to enjoy a greater independence and quality of life through the provision of specially trained dogs. The Charity is working closely with the uniformed services to provide assistance dogs to those injured while on active duty.

More than 1.2 million people in the UK use a wheelchair, and a significant number of those would benefit from a canine partner. The dogs are trained to help with everyday tasks such as opening and shutting doors, unloading the washing machine, picking up dropped items, pressing buttons and switches and getting help in an emergency.

These life transforming dogs also provide practical, physiological, psychological and social benefits including increased independence and confidence as well as increased motivation and self-esteem.

Canine Partners receives no government funding and relies solely on public donations.

For further information visit www.caninepartners.org.uk, email info@caninepartners.org.uk or phone 08456 580480.

Canine Partners, Mill Lane, Heyshott, Midhurst, West Sussex GU29 0ED